中医
临床

Project Editor: Liu Shui & Guo Xiao-li
Book Designer: Li Xi
Cover Designer: Li Xi
Typesetter: Wei Hong-bo

The Clinical Practice of Chinese Medicine

Urticaria

The Clinical Practice of Chinese Medicine

Urticaria

by **Lu Chuan-jian** & **Chen Da-can**

Co-authored with **Huang Yong-jing, Mo Xiu-mei** & **Huang Liang**

Translated by **Wang Juan**
Edited by **Andrea Kurtz**

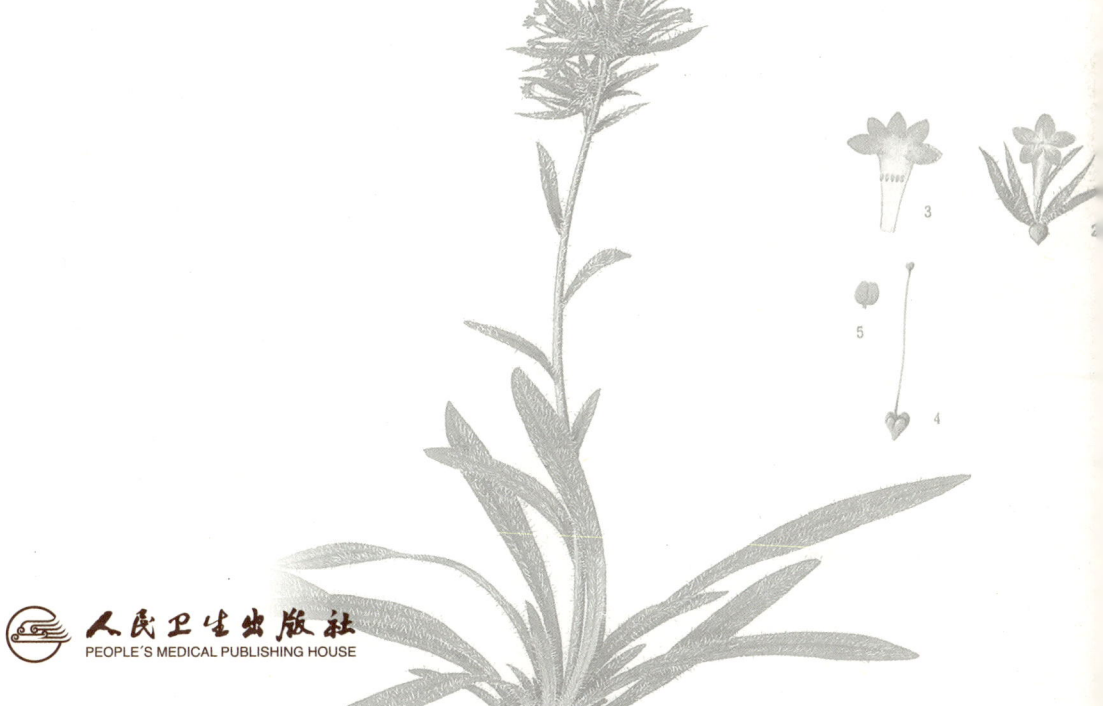

人民卫生出版社
PEOPLE'S MEDICAL PUBLISHING HOUSE

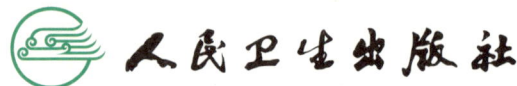

PMPH   PEOPLE'S MEDICAL PUBLISHING HOUSE

www.pmph.com

Book Title: The Clinical Practice of Chinese Medicine: Urticaria
中医临床实用系列：荨麻疹

Contact address: Bldg 3, 3 Qu, Fang Qun Yuan, Fang Zhuang, Beijing 100078, P. R. China, Phone/fax: 86 10 6761 7315, E-mail: pmph@pmph.com

First published: 2007
ISBN: 978-7-117-08533-5/R · 8534

Cataloguing in Publication Data:
A catalog record for this book is available from the
CIP - Database China.

Printed in P. R. China

ISBN 978-7-117-08533-5

9 787117 085335 >

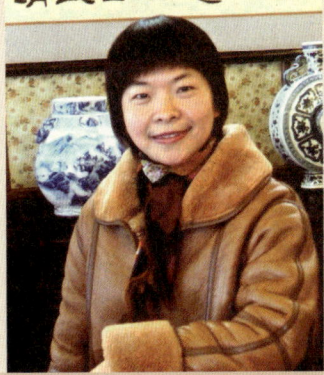

卢传坚 教授

Professor **Lu Chuan-jian** was born in October 1964. She is a Medical Doctor, professor, and state-approved Master's level advisor at the Second Clinical Medicine College of Guangzhou University of Chinese Medicine (also known as the Chinese Medicine Hospital of Guangdong Province). She is also the vice-president of this hospital. In addition, she serves as the vice-president of the Chinese Medicine Diagnosis Specialty Board of the Guangdong Provincial Medicine Association, the standing Director of Clinical Education Board of Advanced Education of Chinese Medicine Association, and as a member of the Dermatology Board of the Guangdong Provincial Medicine Association. She was chosen to be an apprentice of a famous senior physician Professor Shen Yan-nan in the national Master and Apprentice Education Program.

Through her years of clinical practice, teaching, and scientific research she has achieved great curative effects in treating diseases such as psoriasis, eczema, urticaria, cutaneous pruritis, and herpes zoster. She has participated in 11 projects of scientific research on the national, provincial and bureau levels, and has published more than 50 research papers in national or provincial journals, as well as the monograph *Modern-day Treatment to Dermatology & Venereology*. She is the chief editor of *Urticaria, Eczema & Atopic Dermatitis, and Psoriasis & Cutaneous Pruritis*, as part of the *Clinical Practice of Chinese Medicine series*. Professor Lu also participated in the editing and publication of *Diagnosis of Chinese Medicine and Collection of Cases in Dermatology*. She has won 7 clinical and teaching achievement awards.

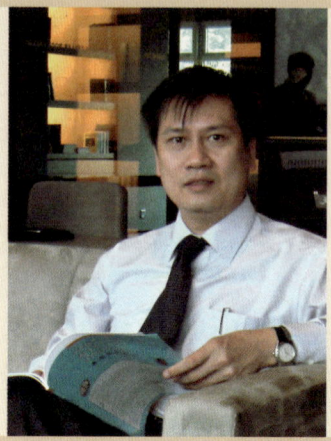

陈达灿 教授

Professor **Chen Da-can** serves as a professor, chief physician, and state-approved Doctoral advisor at the Second Clinical Medicine College of the Guangzhou University of Chinese Medicine (also known as the Chinese Medicine Hospital of Guangdong Province). He is also the vice-president of the Integrated Chinese and Western Medicine Dermatology and Venereology Board, and the vice-president of the Dermatology Branch of the Chinese Medicine Association. Professor Chen is the standing Director of the Guangdong Provincial Medicine Association, as well as the President of the Guangdong Dermatology Board. Through the national Master and Apprentice Education Program he was chosen to be an apprentice of famous senior physicians Professor Xuan Guo-wei and Professor Zhu Liang-chun. In addition, he is the editor of the textbook *Integration of Chinese and Western Medicine in Dermatology and Venereology*, as well as the member of Editorial Committee for both the *Chinese Journal of Integration of Chinese and Western Medicine in Dermatology* and Venereology, and the *New Chinese Medicine journal*.

He has been engaged in clinical practice, teaching, and scientific research since he graduated from the Guangzhou University of Chinese Medicine. Professor Chen specializes in treating diseases such as alopecia, allergic dermatitis, and sexual transmitted diseases. He has a solid foundation in Chinese medical theory and a rich clinical experience, with expertise in the treatment of eczema, urticaria and atopic dermatitis. He has published over 70 research papers in several famous Chinese medical journals and been the chief editor for 7 books including *Clinical Diagnosis and Treatment of Dermatology and Venereology* and *Integration of Chinese and Western Medicine in Surgery*. Professor Chen also participated in the editing and publication of 6 monographs. He has participated in 17 projects of scientific research on the national, provincial and bureau levels, and has won 10 clinical and scientific research achievement awards.

Foreword

Chinese medicine is a broad and profound art of healing. It is a well-established and comprehensive system of medicine with an ancient origin and a long rich history. Throughout the ages, it has made a significant contribution to the prosperity of the Chinese civilization. The system of pattern differentiation and treatment fully reflects the Chinese medical view of health and disease as a holistic concept, the emphasis on the body's ability to regulate itself and adapt to the environment, and the need for individualized treatment. The integration of diseases and syndromes is the consummation of treatment based on pattern differentiation; it fully displays the superior characteristic of this discipline, and has an extensive influence on the development of the art of Chinese medicine.

The intention of this series of books is to introduce accurate Chinese medical diagnosis and treatment of various diseases to overseas readers.

The Chinese edition of *The Clinical Practice of Chinese Medicine* was edited by the Traditional Chinese Medicine Hospital of Guangdong Province (also known as the Second Affiliated Hospital of Guangzhou Chinese Medical University), and published by People's Medical Publishing House. When the series was published in 2000, it was widely accepted in clinical practice due to its originality, distinguishing features, richness in content, completeness, accuracy, and outstanding emphases. This series has become a trademark of standard in the eyes of Chinese and integrative medical practitioners. During the second printing of this series of books, Professor Deng Tie-tao praised, "For a series to be printed a multiple number of times, shows that it is highly regarded and has received excellent reviews." In order to keep up with the constant development of medical science, this series was revised and re-published in 2004 by People's Medical Publishing House. Due to its popularity, it has been reprinted numerous times since.

The English edition of this series of books includes 20 volumes:

✧ *COPD & Asthma*
✧ *Coronary Artery Disease & Hyperlipidemia*
✧ *Stroke & Parkinson's Disease*
✧ *Chronic Gastritis & Irritable Bowel Syndrome*
✧ *Diabetes & Obesity*
✧ *Gout & Rheumatoid Arthritis*
✧ *Menstrual Disorders I: Dysfunctional Uterine Bleeding & Amenorrhea*
✧ *Menstrual Disorders II: Premenstrual Syndrome, Dysmenorrhea & Perimenopause*
✧ *Endometriosis & Uterine Fibroids*
✧ *Pelvic Inflammatory Disease & Miscarriage*
✧ *Postpartum Hypogalactia & Breast Hyperplasia*
✧ *Male & Female Infertility*
✧ *Urticaria*
✧ *Eczema & Atopic Dermatitis*
✧ *Lupus Erythematosus*
✧ *Scleroderma & Dermatomyositis*
✧ *Diseases of the Accessory Organs of the Skin*
✧ *Psoriasis & Cutaneous Pruritis*

✧ *Herpes Zoster & Fungal Skin Infections*
✧ *Pigmentary Disorders of the Skin*

Clinical application varies by individual and by location; when this is combined with the rapid development of medical science, the treatment methods and medicinal dosages may also vary accordingly. When using these books as a reference guide, overseas readers should confirm the formulas and dosages of medicinals according to the individual health condition of the patient, as well as take into account the origin of the Chinese medicinals.

The quotes in these books were taken from various medical literature during the compilation process. We have deleted some of the contents of the original texts for the purpose of uniformity and ease in readability. We ask for the reader's forgiveness and express our respect and gratitude toward the original authors.

Due to the complicated nature of the diagnoses and treatments covered in these books, and the wide range of topics they touch upon, it is inevitable that one may encounter errors while reading through them. We respectively welcome constructive criticism and corrections from our readers.

The clinical practice of medicine changes with the constant development of medical science. The books in this series will be revised regularly to continuously adapt to the development of traditional Chinese medicine.

Editorial Board for the English edition of
The Clinical Practice of Chinese Medicine series
September, 2006

Wu Xian-zhong

Specialist of Integrative Medicine, Academician of Chinese Academy of Engineering, Professor, Tianjin Medical University, Chairman of Tianjin Institute of Acute Abdomen Research on Integrative Medicine

Wang Yong-yan

Specialist of Chinese Internal Medicine, Academician of Chinese Academy of Engineering, Professor and former President of Beijing University of TCM, and Honorary President of China Academy of Chinese Medical Science

Chen Ke-ji

Specialist of Cardiovascular & Aging Diseases, Academician of Chinese Academy of Science, Professor of Medicine, Xiyuan Hospital, and Institute of Aging Medicine, China Academy of Chinese Medical Science, Consultant on Traditional Medicine, WHO

General Coordinator

Lü Yu-bo

Professor & vice-President, Guangzhou University of TCM, President, the Second Teaching Hospital of Guangzhou University of TCM

Editors-in-Chief

Luo Yun-jian

Guangdong Province Entitled Famous Chinese Medicine Physician, Professor of Chinese Internal Medicine, & former vice-President of the Second Teaching Hospital of Guangzhou University of TCM

Liu Mao-cai

Guangdong Province Entitled Famous Chinese Medicine Physician, Professor of Chinese Internal Medicine, & former vice-President of the Second Teaching Hospital of Guangzhou University of TCM, Former Chairman of Institute for Aging Cerebral Diseases, Guangzhou University of TCM

Associate Editors-in-Chief

Xuan Guo-wei

Guangdong Province Entitled Famous Chinese Medicine Physician, Director & Professor, Department of Chinese External Medicine, Guangzhou University of TCM, Former vice-President of the Second Teaching Hospital of Guangzhou University of TCM

Huang Chun-lin

Professor of Chinese Internal Medicine, & former Associate-Director of the Second Institute for Clinical Research, Guangzhou University of TCM

Chen Da-can

Professor of Chinese External Medicine, vice-President of the Second Teaching Hospital of Guangzhou University of TCM

Chen Zhi-qiang

Professor of Chinese External Medicine, Director of the Department of Surgery, vice-President of the Second Teaching Hospital of Guangzhou University of TCM

Feng Wei-bin

Professor of Chinese Internal Medicine, the Second Teaching Hospital of Guangzhou University of TCM

Yang Zhi-min

Professor of Chinese Internal Medicine, vice-President of the Second Teaching Hospital of Guangzhou University of TCM

Lu Chuan-jian

Professor of Chinese External Medicine, vice-President of the Second Teaching Hospital of Guangzhou University of TCM

Zou Xu

Professor of Chinese Internal Medicine, vice-President of the Second Teaching Hospital of Guangzhou University of TCM

Members (Listed alphabetically by name)

Deng Zhao-zhi

Professor of Chinese Internal Medicine, Guangzhou University of TCM

Fan Guan-jie

Professor of Chinese Internal Medicine, Director of Department of Education, the Second Teaching Hospital of Guangzhou University of TCM

Fan Rui-qiang

Professor of Chinese External Medicine, Director of Department of Dermatology, the Second Teaching Hospital of Guangzhou University of TCM

Huang Jian-ling

Professor of Chinese Medicine Gynecology, Director of the First Department of Gynecology, the Second Teaching Hospital of Guangzhou University of TCM

Huang Pei-xin

Professor of Chinese Internal Medicine, the Second Teaching Hospital of Guangzhou University of TCM, Head of the Research Project of Cerebral Disease Treatment on Chinese Internal Medicine, Sponsored by SATCM China

Huang Sui-ping

Professor of Chinese Internal Medicine, Director of Department of Digestion, the Second Teaching Hospital of Guangzhou University of TCM

Li Li-yun

Guangdong Province Entitled Famous Chinese Medicine Physician, Professor of Chinese Medicine Gynecology, the Second Teaching Hospital of Guangzhou University of TCM

Liang Xue-fang

Professor of Chinese Medicine Gynecology, Director of the Third Department of Gynecology, the Second Teaching Hospital of Guangzhou University of TCM

Lin Lin

Professor of Chinese Internal Medicine, Director of Department of Respiratory, the Second Teaching Hospital of Guangzhou University of TCM

Liu Wei-sheng

Master of the National Master and Apprentice Education Program, Professor of Chinese Internal Medicine, the Second Teaching Hospital of Guangzhou University of TCM

Wang Xiao-yun

Professor of Chinese Medicine Gynecology, Director of Department of Gynecology, Head of Teaching Division of Gynecology, the Second Teaching Hospital of Guangzhou University of TCM

Lin Yi

Professor of Mastopathy in Chinese Medicine, the Second Teaching Hospital of Guangzhou University of TCM, Head of the National Key Subject –Mastopathy in Chinese Medicine

Situ Yi

Professor of Chinese Medicine Gynecology, the Second Teaching Hospital of Guangzhou University of TCM, Head of the National Key Subject – Chinese Medicine Gynecology

Sponsored by

The Second Teaching Hospital of Guangzhou University of TCM, also known as **Gongdong Provincial Hospital of TCM**

Preface

Dermatology is a significant component of traditional Chinese medicine. It has an exceedingly rich content due to several thousands of years of accumulated valuable clinical experiences. In the last ten years there have been especially positive developments in the use of traditional Chinese and integrated traditional Chinese and western medicine in the treatment of difficult diseases like eczema, psoriasis, vitiligo, and hair loss. There have also been accomplishments of obvious clinical curative effects, with some already leading international standards.

The authors of this series are all Chinese medical doctors practicing dermatology. They have accumulated abundant experience through years of clinical practice, as well as having published many dermatology text books. Through this compilation process, we have tried to give a detailed introduction to TCM syndrome differentiation and treatments. We have consulted with the editorial board and dermatology specialists to collect advice and suggestions, as well as to summarize their experience of effective treatments. Meanwhile, we have also referred to a large number of related national and international documents that analyze and explore the subject based on current research results. In general, this series is a summarization and refinement of the clinical experience of treating skin diseases with Chinese medicine. It is also our thorough reflections on the key points and challenges of this subject.

Urticaria is the disease that is commonly seen in the

dermatology department. Based on the course of disease, urticaria can be divided into acute and chronic types. Chinese medicine and biomedicine both have satisfying results in the treatment of acute urticaria. However, chronic urticaria has an indefinite and complicated etiology and is hard to cure. It manifests with repeated reoccurrences, and the sudden onset can be severe, with symptoms that can lead to asphyxia and shock, endangering the life of the patient. Therefore preventing and reducing the recurrences of urticaria becomes the challenging clinical task. Fortunately, Chinese medicine is obviously good at achieving that goal. In addition to correlating treatments according to pattern differentiation, proper herbs can be chosen to control infection, eliminate the original cause, and reduce the number of flare-ups.

In this series of books, readers will find an organized and thorough presentation of each disease, including a brief overview, etiology, pathomechanism, Chinese medical treatment using various treatment modalities, prognosis, preventive healthcare practices, case studies, comments from famous physicians, integrative treatment approaches, quotes from classical texts, and modern research.

The **brief overview** offers a general introduction to the biomedical view of the disease.

Discussions of etiology, pathomechanism, and Chinese medical treatment are from the angle of Chinese medicine, and reflect upon the onset, diagnosis, pattern differentiation, and treatment of the disease.

Cases and comments from many famous physicians are collected in the section of clinical experience of renowned physicians.

The chapter on **integrative treatment approaches** emphasizes the advantages of Chinese medical treatments, as well as discussing the proper time for the intervention of biomedicine. To the Western reader, this section presents a clear mode of thinking in terms of the integration of Chinese medicine and biomedicine.

Quotes from classical texts and modern research provide abundant references on these diseases.

This series of books presents a clear description of each disease as well as the key points for diagnosis and treatment using Chinese medicine. These books discuss, in detail, the clinical experience of ancient and modern-day renowned physicians, thereby enabling the practitioner to become more adept at using Chinese medicine in the diagnosis and treatment of common diseases.

In order to ensure a better understanding of the contents of this Chinese medical book series, we have recognized that different readers have different needs and desires.

First, medical professionals, practitioners and students, can read this series for professional study and application, and should have a solid background in the basic theory of Chinese medicine, as well as a mastery of the ingredients and indications of classical formulas. Prior to reading this book, they should also have knowledge of the properly of herbs and combinative contraindications. At the same time, when using the herbs in clinic, practitioners should pay attention to the doses of medicinals and their place of origin. It is fundamental in countries without Chinese herbal medicine, to have a deep understanding of the functions and incompatibilities of the herbs. On the basis of these understandings, one can choose to substitute similar medicinals and formulas to treat illness.

Second, readers who are interested in Chinese medicine should pay attention to the characteristics and advantages of Chinese medicine, and the special methods of Chinese medicine in areas of prognosis and preventive healthcare. In terms of treating patients, if similar symptoms occur, medicine should be prescribed only under the guidance of professional Chinese medical physicians.

We hope that these books will prove to be useful and valuable to all of those involved in the field of Chinese medicine, including practitioners, students, teachers, patients, medical doctors who are interested in Chinese medicine, and anyone who may be seeking answers to their questions about the efficacy of Chinese medicine. Hopefully, this book can help readers gain a deeper understanding of Chinese medical diagnosis and treatment in the field dermatology, as well as build a bridge between Chinese medicine and biomedicine through the discussion of integrative treatment approaches.

Due to the nature of clinical medicine, we apologize for any out-dated or incorrect information that may appear in these books. We hope that readers will not hesitate to offer their comments and suggestions on how to improve the content of this material.

Lu Chuan-jian & Chen Da-can
Guangzhou China
June 2006

Contents

Urticaria

OVERVIEW

Urticaria is a common allergic disease. It manifests on the skin and mucous membranes as temporary inflammation, hyperemia, and fluid exudation. It is caused by various factors that lead to localized edematous damage. There are localized edematous wheals of different sizes; characterized by sudden onset and disappearance. Generally speaking, they last no more than 24 hours and disappear without leaving marks. Urticaria can be accompanied by severe pruritus, burning sensations, and stabbing pain. In severe cases, it can be accompanied by fever. If the digestive system is involved, there can be nausea, vomiting, abdominal pain, and diarrhea. If the larynx and bronchia are involved, there can be laryngeal edema, manifesting as an obstructive sensation in the throat, shortness of breath, chest depression, dyspnea, or asphyxia. On the basis of the course of the disease, urticaria can be divided into two categories: acute and chronic. In the acute type, the onset period can last from several days to 1-2 weeks. In some cases, it will repeatedly reoccur with aggravations over 1-2 months and up to several years. Sometimes this can transform into chronic urticaria. In addition to differentiation based on clinical manifestations, there are different types and categories of urticaria as follows: cold urticaria, heat urticaria, cholinergic urticaria, sunlight urticaria (urticaria solaris), pressure urticaria and water urticaria.

This disease has complicated etiologies and can be caused by internal and external factors including foods, medicines, infections, inhaled substances, physical and chemical factors, inherited factors, endocrine diseases, and mental-emotional stimulations. The pathogenesis can be divided into two categories: allergic reactions and non-allergic reactions. Diagnosis can be easily made according to the typical skin rash characteristics of urticaria. This includes a sudden onset of wheals that disappear without a trace within 24 hours, and are accompanied by pruritus. The specific categories of urticaria should be diagnosed according to their clinical characteristics. Clinical examinations show increased eosinophils in the blood serum. In some cases, the skin scratch test is positive. Patch tests and allergen detection tests can be helpful to look for causative factors. Once these are known, desensitization therapy can be used, and aggravating factors can be avoided in daily life.

Urticaria is treated mainly by internal methods. Since its etiology and pathogenesis are complicated, the treatment principle should be to first seek and remove causative factors, and avoid any kind of inducing factor. Secondly it is necessary to relieve itching and control symptoms. For acute urticaria, H1 receptor antagonists can often be used for control or cure. When urticaria is accompanied by systemic symptoms such as fever, swollen joint pain, abdominal pain, vomiting, diarrhea and dyspnea, corticosteroids can be used early and in full doses as short-term treatments. Prevention of anaphylactic shock and laryngeal edema should be emphasized. Antihistamines are commonly used in the treatment of chronic urticaria. Many other treatment methods can be used, including calcium medications, procaine vein blocking therapy, blood therapy, desensitization therapy, histamine globulin, trasylol, transfer factors, and vitamins. For specific types of urticaria, in addition to using antihistamines, other medications can be used. These include chloroquine for sunlight urticaria, atropine and probanthine for cholinergic urticaria, and doxepin and cyproheptadine for cold urticaria. Aminocaproic acid, histamine globulin and vitamin E can also be used. Artificial urticaria can be treated with hydroxyzine, cinnarizine and doxepin; angioedema can be treated with cromolyn sodium aerosol inhalation, or vaccine-specific desensitization therapy. It is important to note that corticosteroids should not be the first or primary choice for treatment of urticaria, particularly in cases of chronic urticaria.

Urticaria belongs to the category of "habitual rash" (*yǐn zhěn* 瘾疹) and "ghost wind lump" (*guǐ fēng gē da* 鬼风疙瘩).

CHINESE MEDICAL ETIOLOGY AND PATHOMECHANISM

Chinese medicine believes that the onset of urticaria is caused by internal and external factors. The internal causative factor is an intolerant constitution. External etiologies include induction by various sensitizing agents, such as food, medicine, biological products, infected lesions, intestinal parasites, emotional problems, and external invasions of cold and heat evils.

There are many pathogeneses of urticaria. It can be from an external attack and accumulation on the skin with wind-cold, causing disharmony of *ying* and *wei* aspects. Or it can be caused by wind-heat evil attacking the body surface, leading to disharmony of *ying* and *wei* aspects. It can be from improper diet, or intestinal parasites leading to damp-heat in the Intestine and Stomach with an accumulation in the skin and muscular interstitial spaces. It can also be caused by a poor constitution with deficient qi and blood. Qi and blood become consumed due to long-term illness and blood deficiency can engender wind; this causes insecurity of the *wei* aspect due to qi deficiency and wind evil can attack, taking advantage of this weak point. Perhaps from emotional internal damage, dis-regulation of the *Chong* and *Ren* vessels, Liver and Kidney insufficiency, the flesh and skin become malnourished. This engenders wind and dryness, which become depressed in the flesh and skin.

CHINESE MEDICAL TREATMENT

The clinical manifestations of urticaria are complicated. The length of the course of disease can vary, and there are repeated reoccurrences. The treatment should be based on the pattern differentiation according to clinical manifestations and the length of disease course. At present time, treatment of acute urticaria with Chinese medicine is satisfying but treating chronic urticaria is more difficult.

Pattern Differentiation and Treatment

Generally speaking, acute urticaria belongs to an excess pattern and should be treated mainly by the principles of dispelling wind, clearing heat, scattering coldness, cooling blood, resolving toxin or eliminating accumulation of damp-heat in the Intestine and Stomach. Chronic urticaria mainly belongs to a deficiency or stasis pattern and should be treated by the principles of tonifying qi and strengthening the exterior, nourishing blood and dispelling wind, moving blood circulation and freeing the collaterals, strengthening the Spleen and harmonizing the Stomach, and regulating the Chong and Ren vessels.

(1) Wind & Heat Contending

【Syndrome Characteristics】 Red wheals are clustered into geographic patches. The wheals are very hot to the touch. Severe pruritus is aggravated by exposure to heat and relieved by cold. It can be accompanied by a slight fever and aversion to wind, Heart vexation, thirst, pharyngeal congestion, a red tongue body with a thin, yellow or scanty coat, and a superficial and rapid pulse.

【Treatment Principle】 Clear heat and relieve the exterior, calm wind and relieve itching.

【Commonly Used Medicinals】 *Jīn yín huā* (Flos Lonicerae Japonicae) and *lián qiào* (Fructus Forsythiae) can be used to clear heat and release the exterior. *Dàn zhú yè* (Herba Lophatheri), *niú bàng zǐ* (Fructus Arctii), and *lú gēn* (Rhizoma Phragmitis) can be used to drain heat downward. *Niú bàng zǐ* (Fructus Arctii), *bò hé* (Herba Menthae) and *chán tuì* (Periostracum Cicadae) can be used to calm wind and release exterior.

【Representative Formula】 Modified *Yín Qiào Sǎn* （银翘散）

【Ingredients】

金银花	jīn yín huā	15g	Flos Lonicerae Japonicae
连翘	lián qiào	15g	Fructus Forsythiae
淡竹叶	dàn zhú yè	10g	Herba Lophatheri
鱼腥草	yú xīng cǎo	20g	Herba Houttuyniae
牛蒡子	niú bàng zǐ	10g	Fructus Arctii
薄荷（后下）	bò hé	5g	Herba Menthae (decoct later)
荆芥	jīng jiè	10g	Herba Schizonepetae
浮萍	fú píng	15g	Herba Spirodelae
蝉蜕	chán tuì	10g	Periostracum Cicadae
芦根	lú gēn	15g	Rhizoma Phragmitis
甘草	gān cǎo	5g	Radix et Rhizoma Glycyrrhizae

Decoct in 500 ml of water until 100 ml of the decoction is left. Take warm, twice a day.

【Formula Analysis】 *Jīn yín huā* (Flos Lonicerae Japonicae) and *lián qiào* (Fructus Forsythiae) work as the chief herbs. They are pungent in flavor and cool in property, therefore they dispel pathogenic factors from exterior, clear heat and resolve toxin in addition to avoiding foulness by being fragrant and aromatic. *Niú bàng zǐ* (Fructus Arctii) and *bò hé* (Herba Menthae) are pungent in flavor and cool in property, *jīng jiè* (Herba Schizonepetae), *fú píng* (Herba Spirodelae) and *chán tuì* (Periostracum Cicadae) are pungent in flavor and slightly warm in property. These work as the deputies to assist the chief herbs to dispel pathogenic factors from exterior, clear heat, and remove skin rashes. *Yú xīng cǎo* (Herba Houttuyniae), *lú gēn* (Rhizoma Phragmitis) and *dàn zhú yè* (Herba Lophatheri) work as the assistants to clear the Lung, disinhibit water and remove skin rashes. *Gān cǎo* (Radix et Rhizoma Glycyrrhizae) works as the envoy to harmonize the actions of the other herbs, and to protect the Stomach. There are two characteristics of this prescription. The first is that a few pungent and warm herbs assist pungent and cool herbs in order to dispel pathogenic factors from exterior, and at the same time keep to the principle of using pungent and coolness. The second is that the combination of dispel wind evil herbs with clear heat herbs can resolve toxin and avoid foulness by using aromatic properties that clear and dispel.

【Modifications】 For cough with yellow phlegm, add *sāng bái pí* (Cortex Mori) 15g and *xìng rén* (Semen Armeniacae Dulcis) 10g to clear heat and resolve phlegm.

For dry stool, add *zǐ cǎo* (Radix Arnebiae) 15g and *dōng guā rén* (Semen Benincasae) 15g to cool the blood, moisten bowels and promote bowel movement.

For vexation, add *dì gǔ pí* (Cortex Lycii) 10g and *zhēn zhū mǔ* (Concha Margaritifera) 30g to clear heat, cool blood and relieve restlessness.

For sore throat, add *bǎn lán gēn* (Radix Isatidis) 20g and *shān dòu gēn* (Radix et Rhizoma Sophorae Tonkinensis) 5g to resolve toxin and relieve sore throat.

(2) Wind & Cold Fettering the Exterior

【Syndrome Characteristics】 Wheals are light red or the color of white porcelain. They are aggravated by exposure to wind or cold water and relieved by warmth. Accompanying are aversion to wind and cold, no thirst, a slightly red tongue, a thin and white coat, and a superficial and tight pulse.

【Treatment Principle】 Expel wind and resolve cold, regulate *ying* and *wei* aspects.

【Commonly Used Medicinals】 *Guì zhī* (Ramulus Cinnamomi), *má huáng* (Herba Ephedrae), *sū yè* (Folium Perillae), *fáng fēng* (Radix Saposhnikoviae), *jīng jiè suì* (Spica Schizonepetae), and *shēng jiāng*

(Rhizoma Zingiberis Recens) expel wind and cold.

【**Representative Formula**】 Modified *Guì Zhī Má Huáng Gè Bàn Tāng* (桂枝麻黄各半汤)

【**Ingredients**】

桂技	guì zhī	12g	Ramulus Cinnamomi
麻黄	má huáng	6g	Herba Ephedrae
白芍	bái sháo	15g	Radix Paeoniae Alba
大枣	dà zǎo	6	Fructus Jujubae
苏叶	sū yè	12g	Folium Perillae
防风	fáng fēng	12g	Radix Saposhnikoviae
荆芥穗	jīng jiè suì	15g	Spica Schizonepetae
杏仁	xìng rén	12g	Semen Armeniacae Dulcis
生姜	shēng jiāng	3pieces	Rhizoma Zingiberis Recens
甘草	gān cǎo	3g	Radix et Rhizoma Glycyrrhizae

Decoct in 500 ml of water until 100 ml of the decoction is left. Take warm, twice a day.

【**Formula Analysis**】 *Guì zhī* (Ramulus Cinnamomi) and *má huáng* (Herba Ephedrae) work as the chief herbs to calm wind, release the exterior and dispel cold. *Fáng fēng* (Radix Saposhnikoviae) and *jīng jiè suì* (Spica Schizonepetae) dispel wind and relieve itching; *bái sháo* (Radix Paeoniae Alba) and *dà zǎo* (Fructus Jujubae) regulate the *ying* and *wei* aspects and work as the deputies. They assist *sū yè* (Folium Perillae), *xìng rén* (Semen Armeniacae Dulcis), and *shēng jiāng* (Rhizoma Zingiberis Recens) to diffuse the Lung and dispel cold. *Gān cǎo* (Radix et Rhizoma Glycyrrhizae) works as the envoy to harmonize the actions of the other herbs. The combination of *má huáng* (Herba Ephedrae) and *guì zhī* (Ramulus Cinnamomi) can not only open the muscular interstitial spaces from depressed *wei qi* but can also expel depressed *ying* in order to harmonize the *ying* and *wei*. This prescription has a tonifying function accompanied by expelling and astringing functions, as well as a dispelling action. It simultaneously deals with the evil and the right, and regulates both the yin and the yang.

【Modifications】

For yang deficiency aggravated by cold, remove *jīng jiè suì* (Spica Schizonepetae), and add *xiān líng pí* (Herba Epimedii) 15g, *bái zhú* (Rhizoma Atractylodis Macrocephalae) 10g and *huáng qí* (Radix Astragali) 20g, so as to warm yang and dispel coldness, boost qi and consolidate the exterior.

For ice-coldness of the four limbs, add *dāng guī* (Radix Angelicae Sinensis) 15g and *lù jiǎo jiāo* (Colla Cornus Cervi) 10g (melted) to nourish the blood and free blood vessels.

For profuse sweating induced by wind, remove *má huáng* (Herba Ephedrae), and add *lóng gǔ* (Os Draconis) 30g (decocted first) and *má huáng gēn* (Radix et Rhizoma Ephedrae) 10g to consolidate the exterior and relieve profuse sweating.

(3) Stomach & Intestine Damp-Heat

【Syndrome Characteristics】 Wheals are bright red and arise from improper diet. They are accompanied mainly by abdominal pain, diarrhea, vomiting, chest oppression, unformed and sluggish stool, a red tongue body with a yellow and greasy coat, and a rapid or soggy, rapid pulse.

【Treatment Principle】 Clear the Intestine and drain dampness, dispel wind and relieve itching.

【Commonly Used Medicinals】 *Zhǐ shí* (Fructus Aurantii Immaturus), *hòu pò* (Cortex Magnoliae Officinalis), *tǔ fú líng* (Rhizoma Smilacis Glabrae), *mián yīn chén* (Herba Artemisiae Scopariae), *jīn yín huā* (Flos Lonicerae Japonicae) and *bù zhā yè* (Microcoris Folium) clear the Intestine and drain dampness; *sū yè* (Folium Perillae) and *fáng fēng* (Radix Saposhnikoviae) dispel wind and relieve itching.

【Representative Formula】 Modified *Tǔ Fú Yīn Chén Tāng* （土茯茵

陈汤）

【Ingredients】

土茯苓	tǔ fú líng	20g	Rhizoma Smilacis Glabrae
绵茵陈	mián yīn chén	20g	Herba Artemisiae Scopariae
金银花	jīn yín huā	15g	Flos Lonicerae Japonicae
火炭母	huǒ tàn mǔ	20g	Polygonum chinensis
布渣叶	bù zhā yè	15g	Microcoris Folium
山楂	shān zhā	20g	Fructus Crataegi
苏叶	sū yè	10g	Folium Perillae
枳实	zhǐ shí	10g	Fructus Aurantii Immaturus
厚朴	hòu pò	10g	Cortex Magnoliae Officinalis
连翘	lián qiào	10g	Fructus Forsythiae
甘草	gān cǎo	5g	Radix et Rhizoma Glycyrrhizae

Decoct in 500 ml of water until 100 ml of the decoction is left. Take warm, twice a day.

【Formula Analysis】 *Tǔ fú líng* (Rhizoma Smilacis Glabrae) and *mián yīn chén* (Herba Artemisiae Scopariae) clear heat and drain dampness; *jīn yín huā* (Flos Lonicerae Japonicae) and *lián qiào* (Fructus Forsythiae) calm wind, clear heat and resolve toxin. Together these work as the chief herbs. *Huǒ tàn mǔ* (Polygonum Chinensis) and *bù zhā yè* (Microcoris Folium) work as the deputies to help the chief herbs clear and drain damp-heat in the Intestine and Stomach. These are assisted by *shān zhā* (Fructus Crataegi), *sū yè* (Folium Perillae), *zhǐ shí* (Fructus Aurantii Immaturus) and *hòu pò* (Cortex Magnoliae Officinalis) in order to promote digestion, move qi and remove stagnated food. *Gān cǎo* (Radix et Rhizoma Glycyrrhizae) works as the envoy to harmonize the actions of the other herbs and to protect the Stomach. This prescription has the main functions of clearing heat and draining dampness, at the same time it moves qi, and promotes digestion to relieve food stagnation. It can transform dampness and regulate qi to relieve symptoms.

【Modifications】

For parasite-induced malnutrition, add *shǐ jūn zǐ ròu* (Fructus Quisqualis) 15g, *wū méi ròu* (Fructus Mume) 9g and *bīng láng* (Semen Arecae) 30g to expel parasites.

For constipation, add *dà huáng* (Radix et Rhizoma Rhei) 6g (decocted at the end) to relax the bowels and purge heat.

(4) Toxic Heat Blazing in the *Ying* Aspect

【Syndrome Characteristics】 This is characterized by a sudden onset, with big patches of red wheals. In severe cases it can spread over the whole body or coagulate into geographic patches. There is severe pruritus accompanied by a high fever, aversion to cold, thirst with a preference for cold drinks, a flushed complexion, red eyes, vexation, constipation, scanty red urine, a red tongue body with a yellow or yellow-dry coat, and a flooding and rapid pulse.

【Treatment Principle】 Clear the *ying* aspect and cool the blood, resolve toxin and relieve itching.

【Commonly Used Medicinals】 *Shuǐ niú jiǎo* (Cornu Bubali), *shēng dì* (Radix Rehmanniae Recens), *xuán shēn* (Radix Scrophulariae), *chì sháo* (Radix Paeoniae Rubra) and *dān pí* (Cortex Moutan) can be used to clear heat and resolve toxin. *Lú gēn* (Rhizoma Phragmitis) and *huáng qín* (Radix Scutellariae) can be used to clear heat and drain dampness. *Zǐ cǎo* (Radix Arnebiae), *chán yī* (Periostracum Cicadae) and *jīng jiè* (Herba Schizonepetae) can be used to calm wind and relieve itching.

【Representative Formula】 *Fù Fāng Shuǐ Niú Jiǎo Tāng* （复方水牛角汤）

【Ingredients】

水牛角 （先煎）	shuǐ niú jiǎo	30g	Cornu Bubali (decoct first)
生地	shēng dì	20g	Radix Rehmanniae Recens
鱼腥草	yú xīng cǎo	20g	Herba Houttuyniae
紫草	zǐ cǎo	20g	Radix Arnebiae
蝉衣	chán yī	10g	Periostracum Cicadae

黄芩	huáng qín	12g	Radix Scutellariae
丹皮	dān pí	12g	Cortex Moutan
玄参	xuán shēn	15g	Radix Scrophulariae
生石膏	shēng shí gāo	20g	Gypsum Fibrosum (raw)
赤芍	chì sháo	15g	Radix Paeoniae Rubra ·
芦根	lú gēn	15g	Rhizoma Phragmitis
甘草	gān cǎo	5g	Radix et Rhizoma Glycyrrhizae

Decoct in 500 ml of water until 100 ml of the decoction is left. Take warm, twice a day.

【Formula Analysis】 *Shuǐ niú jiǎo* (Cornu Bubali), *shēng dì* (Radix Rehmanniae Recens), *zǐ cǎo* (Radix Arnebiae), *dān pí* (Cortex Moutan), and *chì sháo* (Radix Paeoniae Rubra) work as the chief herbs to clear heat and cool blood, resolve toxin and remove wheals. *Yú xīng cǎo* (Herba Houttuyniae), *huáng qín* (Radix Scutellariae), *shēng shí gāo* (raw Gypsum Fibrosum), and *lú gēn* (Rhizoma Phragmitis) act as the deputies to clear the Lung and purge heat in order to help the chief herbs to clear heat and resolve toxin. Assisting are *chán yī* (Periostracum Cicadae) to calm wind, clear heat and relieve itching, *xuán shēn* (Radix Scrophulariae) to cool the blood, nourish yin, resolve toxin, and promote eruption. *Gān cǎo* (Radix et Rhizoma Glycyrrhizae) works as the envoy to harmonize the action of the other herbs and to protect the Stomach. This prescription has the function of clearing *ying* and cooling blood, resolving toxin and relieving itching. These herbs in large dosages clear heat, purge the Lung and cool blood. They assist with *xuán shēn* (Radix Scrophulariae) to cool the blood and nourishing yin, resolve toxin and promoting eruption, and with *chán yī* (Periostracum Cicadae) to calm wind, promote eruption and relieve itching.

【Modifications】

For high fever with red complexion, add *shēng shí gāo* (Gypsum Fibrosom, raw) 40-60g, *jīn yín huā* (Flos Lonicerae Japonicae) 20g and *pú gōng yīng* (Herba Taraxaci) 20g so as to strengthen the function of clearing heat, purging fire and resolving toxin.

For thirst, add *zhī mǔ* (Rhizoma Anemarrhenae) 10g and *huā fěn* (Radix Trichosanthis) 10g to clear heat and nourish yin.

For constipation, add *dà huáng* (Radix et Rhizoma Rhei) 9g to relax the bowels and purge heat.

For sore throat, add *niú bàng zǐ* (Fructus Arctii) 9g, *shè gān* (Rhizoma Belamcandae) 12g and *jié gěng* (Radix Platycodonis) 9g to relieve sore throat and resolve toxin.

(5) *Wei* & Exterior Not Consolidated

【Syndrome Characteristics】 This is characterized by numerous skin rashes, ranging in size from the head of a needle to a lima bean. They rarely coagulate into patches. Nevertheless, the wheals frequently occur in groups when the patient sweats from wind exposure, or has an exterior deficiency with aversion to wind. There is endless pruritus, aversion to wind with spontaneous sweating, a slight red tongue body with thin white or scanty coating and a deep and thready pulse.

【Treatment Principle】 Consolidate the exterior and dispel wind.

【Commonly Used Medicinals】 *Huáng qí* (Radix Astragali) and *bái zhú* (Rhizoma Atractylodis Macrocephalae) boost qi and consolidate the exterior. *Fáng fēng* (Radix Saposhnikoviae) and *jiāng cán* (Bombyx Batryticatus) dispel wind and relieve itching. *Wū méi* (Fructus Mume), *duàn mǔ lì* (Concha Ostreae) (calcined) astringe qi and consolidate the exterior.

【Representative Formula】 Modified *Yù Píng Fēng Sǎn* （玉屏风散）
【Ingredients】

黄芪	huáng qí	30g	Radix Astragali
防风	fáng fēng	15g	Radix Saposhnikoviae
白术	bái zhú	10g	Rhizoma Atractylodis Macrocephalae
乌梅	wū méi	20g	Fructus Mume

煅牡蛎（先煎）	duàn mǔ lì	20g	Concha Ostreae (calcined)(decoct first)
白芍	bái sháo	15g	Radix Paeoniae Alba
茯苓	fú líng	15g	Poria
乌豆衣	wū dòu yī	15g	Spermodermis Phaseoli Radiati
熟地黄	shú dì huáng	15g	Radix Rehmanniae Praeparata
山茱萸	shān zhū yú	15g	Fructus Corni
炙甘草	zhì gān cǎo	5g	Radix et Rhizoma Glycyrrhizae Praeparata cum Melle

Decoct in 500 ml of water until 100 ml of the decoction is left. Take warm, twice a day.

【Formula Analysis】 *Huáng qí* (Radix Astragali) is sweet in flavor and warm in property. It internally tonifies the Spleen and Lung *qi*, and externally consolidates the exterior and relieves profuse sweating. *Bái zhú* (Rhizoma Atractylodis Macrocephalae) and *fú líng* (Poria) strengthen the Spleen and tonify qi. With *huáng qí* (Radix Astragali) they act as the chief herbs. *Wū méi* (Fructus Mume), *shān zhū yú* (Fructus Corni) and *duàn mǔ lì* (Concha Ostreae calcined) astringe qi and consolidate the exterior; *bái sháo* (Radix Paeoniae Alba), *wū dòu yī* (Spermodermis Phaseoli Radiati) and *shú dì huáng* (Radix Rehmanniae Praeparata) nourish the blood and act as the deputies. Assisting is *fáng fēng* (Radix Saposhnikoviae) to expel wind and relieve itching from the exterior. *Zhì gān cǎo* (prepared Radix et Rhizoma Glycyrrhizae) works as the envoy to warm Middle Jiao and strengthen the Spleen. This prescription is characterized by predominance of herbs that tonify the qi and consolidate the exterior. There are assistant herbs that nourish blood and astringe. They are combined with herbs, used in small amounts, that expel wind and release the exterior. Therefore this prescription can dispel and tonify - it can disperse evils without damaging the right *qi*.

【Modifications】

For profuse sweating, add *fú xiǎo mài* (Fructus Tritici Levis) 15g and *wǔ wèi zǐ* (Fructus Schisandrae Chinensis) 10g to consolidate the exterior and relieve profuse sweating.

For aversion to cold and wind, add *guì zhī* (Ramulus Cinnamomi) 9g and *má huáng* (Herba Ephedrae) 3g to calm wind and dispel cold.

(6) Qi & Blood Depleted and Deficiency

【Syndrome Characteristics】 Wheals are pale red or the same color with the skin. They repeatedly reoccur, lingering over several months or years without cure. They are aggravated by fatigue and are accompanied by dizziness, mental fatigue, pale complexion, tiredness, lack of strength, insomnia; a slight red tongue body with a thin white or scanty coating, and a thready and moderate pulse.

【Treatment Principle】 Tonify qi and blood.

【Commonly Used Medicinals】 *Dăng shēn* (Radix Codonopsis), *bái zhú* (Rhizoma Atractylodis Macrocephalae) and *fú líng* (Poria) tonify qi. *Chăo bái sháo* (Stir-fried Radix Paeoniae Alba) and *shú dì* (Radix Rehmanniae Praeparata) nourish blood.

【Representative Formula】 Modified *Bā Zhēn Tāng* （八珍汤）

【Ingredients】

党参	dǎng shēn	15g	Radix Codonopsis
白术	bái zhú	12g	Rhizoma Atractylodis Macrocephalae
茯苓	fú líng	12g	Poria
炒白芍	chǎo bái sháo	9g	Stir-fried Radix Paeoniae Alba (stir-fried)
熟地	shú dì	12g	Radix Rehmanniae Praeparata
川芎	chuān xiōng	6g	Rhizoma Chuanxiong
甘草	gān cǎo	6g	Radix et Rhizoma Glycyrrhizae
阿胶（另烊）	ē jiāo	15g	Colla Corii Asini (dissolved)

Decoct in 500 ml of water until 100 ml of the decoction is left. Take warm twice day.

【Formula Analysis】 *Dăng shēn* (Radix Codonopsis) strengthens the Spleen and tonifies qi, *shú dì* (Radix Rehmanniae Praeparata) tonifies essence and blood. These act as the chief herbs. *Bái zhú* (Rhizoma Atractylodis Macrocephalae) and *fú líng* (Poria) strengthen the Spleen and drain dampness. They are assisted by *dǎng shēn* (Radix Codonopsis) to tonify the qi and Spleen, *ē jiāo* (Colla Corii Asini) and *bái sháo* (Radix Paeoniae Alba) to nourish blood and harmonize *ying*, and *shú dì* (Radix Rehmanniae Praeparata) to tonify yin and blood. All together they are the deputies. *Chuān xiōng* (Rhizoma Chuanxiong) assists by activating blood circulation and moving qi in order to tonify without stagnating. *Gān cǎo* (Radix et Rhizoma Glycyrrhizae) acts as the envoy to tonify qi, regulate the Middle Jiao, and harmonize the actions of the other herbs. In order to avoid stagnation, this prescription has the function of tonifying qi and nourishing blood by using a tonification method accompanied by a moving method.

【Modifications】

For unformed stool, remove *shú dì* (Radix Rehmanniae Praeparata), and add *fú líng* (Poria) 20g and *huái shān yào* (Rhizoma Dioscoreae) 20g to strengthen Spleen and drain dampness.

For severe pruritus, add *fáng fēng* (Radix Saposhnikoviae) 10g, *mǔ lì* (Concha Ostreae) 30g, and *cì jí lí* (Fructus Tribuli) 10g to dispel wind and relieve itching.

For vexation and palpitation, add *mài mén dōng* (Radix Ophiopogonis) 10g and *tài zǐ shēn* (Radix Pseudostellariae) 20g to nourish yin and resolve restlessness.

For night sweats, add *fú xiǎo mài* (Fructus Tritici Levis) 15g to consolidate the exterior and astringe profuse sweating.

For profuse dreaming at night, add *suān zǎo rén* (Semen Ziziphi Spinosae) 30g to nourish the Heart and calm the spirit.

(7) *Chong* & *Ren* Not Regulated

【Syndrome Characteristics】 Wheals are light red and spread mainly on the lower abdomen, lumbar-sacral region and thighs. They are aggravated during the pre-menstrual period and relieved after menstruation. They are often accompanied by irregular menstruation and dysmenorrhea. The tongue body is normal or slightly red, with a thin white or scanty coat. The pulse is wiry and thready or wiry and slippery.

【Treatment Principle】 Regulate the *Chong* and *Ren* vessels.

【Commonly Used Medicinals】 *Xiān máo* (Rhizoma Curculiginis) and *xiān líng pí* (Herba Epimedii) tonify the Kidney yang. *Tù sī zǐ* (Semen Cuscutae) and *nǔ zhēn zǐ* (Fructus Ligustri Lucidi) nourish the Kidney *yin*. *Hàn lián cǎo* (Herba Ecliptae) cools the blood and activates blood circulation. *Dāng guī* (Radix Angelicae Sinensis), *chuān xiōng* (Radix Angelicae Sinensis) and *yì mǔ cǎo* (Herba Leonuri) nourish and move the blood.

【Representative Formula】 Modified *Sì Wù Tāng* with *Er Xiān Tāng* (四物汤合二仙汤)

【Ingredients】

仙茅	xiān máo	6g	Rhizoma Curculiginis
当归	dāng guī	6g	Radix Angelicae Sinensis
川芎	chuān xiōng	6g	Rhizoma Chuanxiong
仙灵脾	xiān líng pí	12g	Herba Epimedii
菟丝子	tù sī zǐ	15g	Semen Cuscutae
女贞子	nǔ zhēn zǐ	15g	Fructus Ligustri Lucidi
旱莲草	hàn lián cǎo	15g	Herba Ecliptae
丹参	dān shēn	15g	Radix et Rhizoma Salviae Miltiorrhizae
牛膝	niú xī	9g	Radix Achyranthis Bidentatae
益母草	yì mǔ cǎo	9g	Herba Leonuri

Decoct in 500 ml of water until 100 ml of the decoction is left. Take warm, twice a day.

【Formula Analysis】 *Xiān máo* (Rhizoma Curculiginis) and *xiān líng pí* (Herba Epimedii) warm the Kidney *yang*; *dāng guī* (Radix Angelicae Sinensis) nourishes and harmonizes the blood. Together they work as the chief herbs. *Tù sī zǐ* (Semen Cuscutae), *nǔ zhēn zǐ* (Fructus Ligustri Lucidi) and *hàn lián cǎo* (Herba Ecliptae) nourish Kidney *yin*, and help the chief herbs to nourish the blood and *yin*, and regulate the *Chong* and *Ren* vessels. They work as the deputies. *Dān shēn* (Radix et Rhizoma Salviae Miltiorrhizae), *chuān xiōng* (Radix Angelicae Sinensis) and *yì mǔ cǎo* (Herba Leonuri) assist to nourish and move the blood, in order to tonify without stagnating. *Niú xī* (Radix Achyranthis Bidentatae) tonifies the Liver and Kidney, and leads the actions of the other herbs downward. It is the envoy. The prescription has the function of strengthening qi and blood, and regulating the *Chong* and *Ren* vessels. It does this by tonifying and moving both the yin and yang aspects.

【Modifications】

For dysmenorrhea, add *sān qī* (Radix et Rhizoma Notoginseng) 6g and *jī xuè téng* (Caulis Spatholobi) 15g to strengthen the actions of moving blood and relieving pain.

For scanty, pale red, and irregular menstruation, add *sāng jì shēng* (Herba Taxilli) 20g and *ē jiāo* (Colla Corii Asini) 15g to tonify the Kidney and nourish blood.

For stubborn skin rashes with severe pruritus, add *quán chóng* (Scorpio) 3-6g, *gōu téng* (Ramulus Uncariae Cum Uncis) 12g, and *bái jí lí* (Fructus Tribuli) 12g to dispel wind, open the channels and relieve itching.

For irritability and restlessness, add *yù jīn* (Radix Curcumae) 15g, *chái hú* (Radix Bupleuri) 10g and *bái sháo* (Radix Paeoniae Alba) 10g to course the Liver, resolve constraint, nourish blood and harmonize the *ying*.

Additional Treatment Modalities

1. CHINESE PATENT MEDICINE

1) *Yù Píng Fēng Kē Lì* (玉屏风颗粒)

Take 5g each time, 3 times a day. This is indicated for a pattern differentiated as chronic urticaria from instability of *wei qi*.

2) *Liù Wèi Dì Huáng Wán* （六味地黄丸）

Take 6g each time, 2 times a day. This is indicated for a pattern differentiated as chronic urticaria from heat in the blood due to yin deficiency.

3) *Bā Zhēn Hé Jì* （八珍合剂）

Take 3.5g each time, 2 times a day. This is indicated for a pattern differentiated as chronic urticaria from deficiency of qi and blood.

4) *Wū Shé Zhǐ Yǎng Wán* （乌蛇止痒丸）

Take half a bag (60 granules) each time, 2 times a day. This is indicated for stubborn urticaria.

2. ACUPUNCTURE AND MOXIBUSTION

(1) Acupuncture Using Filiform Needle

1) Point Selection Along the Course of Channels

【Point Selection】

For wind evil that tends to invade the *yang* channels, select DU 14 (*dà zhuǐ*), SP 10 (*xuè hǎi*) and ST 36 (*zú sān lǐ*).

For dampness evil that tends to invade the Spleen channel, select BL 20 (*pí shù*), LI 11 (*qū chí*) and ST 36 (*zú sān lǐ*).

For blood-dryness causing wind and tending to invade the Liver channel, select SP 6 (*sān yīn jiāo*), SP 10 (*xuè hǎi*) and LV 2 (*xíng jiān*).

【Manipulation】 Use supplementation methods for deficiency patterns, and drainage methods for excess patterns. After the arrival of qi, retain needles for 10-15 minutes. Treat one time every one to two days.

2) Selection of Local Points

【Point Selection】

For skin rashes on the head and face, select SJ 23 (*sī zhú kōng*), EX-

HN 8 (*yíng xiāng*), and GB 20 (*fēng chí*).

For skin rashes on the abdomen, select RN 12 (*zhōng wǎn*).

For skin rashes on the lumbar area, select BL 13 (*fèi shù*) and BL 23 (*shèn shù*).

For skin rashes on the lower limbs, select ST 32(*fú tù*), GB 31 (*fēng shì*), ST 36 (*zú sān lǐ*) and BL 40 (*wěi zhōng*).

【Manipulation】 Use supplementation methods for deficiency patterns, and drainage methods for excess patterns. After the arrival of qi, retain needles for 10 - 15 minutes. Treat one time every one to two days.

3) Point Selection According to Etiology

【Point Selection】

For wind-heat evil, select DU 14 (*dà zhuī*), GB 20 (*fēng chí*), DU 20 (*bǎi huì*), and BL 40 (*wěi zhōng*).

For disharmony of the Intestine and Stomach, select BL 25 (*dà cháng shù*), LI 4 (*hé gǔ*), and ST 36 (*zú sān lǐ*).

【Manipulation】 Use supplementation methods for deficiency patterns, and drainage methods for excess patterns. After the arrival of qi, retain needles for 10 - 15 minutes. Treat one time every one to two days.

4) Experiential Point Selection

【Point Selection】 DU 14 (*dà zhuī*).

【Manipulation】 The depth of insertion is 1.5 cun. The method used is a drainage technique with a large amplitude of rotation. There is no needle retention. Treatment is 1 time per day. This is indicated for acute urticaria.

【Point Selection】 BL 25 (*dà cháng shù*).

【Manipulation】 The method used is a supplementation technique. Retain needles for 30 minutes after the arrival of qi. Manipulate the needles 3-5 times during the retention. Treat 1 time each day. This is indicated for chronic urticaria.

5) Combination of Acupuncture & Bleeding

【Point Combination】

DU 14	dà zhuī	大椎
SJ 10	tiān jǐng	天井
Ambi-SP 10	xuè hǎi	血海
Ambi-GB 39	xuán zhōng	悬钟
Ambi-LI 11	qū chí	曲池
PC 3	qū zé	曲泽
BL 40	wěi zhōng	委中

【Manipulation】 Use an even supplementation and drainage method. After the arrival of qi, retain needles for 5 minutes. After withdrawing the needles, prick PC 3 (*qū zé*) and BL 40 (*wěi zhōng*) and quickly squeeze the skin around the points to get a few drops of blood. Treat 1 time each day. This is indicated for chronic urticaria and cholinergic urticaria.

(2) Moxibustion

【Point Combination】

LI 4	hé gǔ	合谷
LI 11	qū chí	曲池
LV 2	xíng jiān	行间
ST 36	zú sān lǐ	足三里
SP 10	xuè hǎi	血海
SP 6	sān yīn jiāo	三阴交

【Manipulation】 Cut fresh ginger into slices for external application on the points. Use 3-5 moxa-cones for each acupoint. Treat 1 time each day. This is indicated for chronic urticaria and cold urticaria.

(3) External Application on the Umbilicus

【Manipulation】 After sterilizing the umbilicus, use a proper quantity of modified *Yù Píng Fēng Sǎn* (*huáng qí* [Radix Astragali] 30g, *fáng fēng* [Radix Saposhnikoviae] 15g, *bái zhú* [Rhizoma Atractylodis Macrocephalae] 15g , *wū méi* [Fructus Mume] 30g , *jīng jiè* [Herba Schizonepetae] 15g , and *bīng piàn* [Borneolum Syntheticum] 3g , grinded into powder) to fill the umbilicus. Alternatively, mix a modified *Yù Píng Fēng Sǎn* 10g with ground benadryl hydrochloride 50g to fill the umbilicus. Fix it with a sticky preparation of *Fū Jí Níng* (肤疾宁) or a common adhesive fabric. Change the dressing 1 time each day. A course of treatment is 7 days. This is indicated for chronic urticaria.

(4) Ear Acupuncture

1) Ear Acupuncture Therapy

【**Point Combination**】

Lung	CO 14	fèi	肺

And the corresponding parts of the skin lesion.

【**Point Modification**】

For cold urticaria, add GV 17 (*nǎo hù*), Occiput and Sympathetic.

For wind-heat urticaria, add Heart and Liver.

For cholinergic urticaria, add Sympathetic, Adrenal gland, and the Anti-anaphylaxis point.

For protein peptone urticaria, add BL 25 (*dà cháng shù*) and Stomach.

For blood serum disease urticaria, add Heart, Kidney and Shenmen.

【**Manipulation**】 Use a draining method. Retain the needles for 30 minutes. Treat 1 time per day.

2) Ear Acupuncture with Intradermal Needle Therapy

【**Point Combination**】

lung	CO 14	fèi	肺
adrenal gland	TG 2p	shèn shàng xiàn	肾上腺
shenmen	TF 4	shén mén	神门

And the corresponding parts of the skin lesion.

【Manipulation】 Choose 2-3 points each time per ear. Sterilize the points with the routine method, then insert a press-tack needle, and fix it with an adhesive. Retain the needles for 72 hours. Wait 3-4 days and then repeat.

3. EXTERNAL APPLICATION

1) External Wash:

【Prescription】

荆芥	jīng jiè	30g	Herba Schizonepetae
防风	fáng fēng	30g	Radix Saposhnikoviae
川芎	chuān xiōng	20g	Rhizoma Chuanxiong
苏叶	sū yè	20g	Folium Perillae
黄精	huáng jīng	30g	Rhizoma Polygonati
蛇床子	shé chuáng zǐ	30g	Fructus Cnidii

Decoct with water and wash over the skin lesions. This is indicated for chronic urticaria.

2) External Application:

1% *bò hé* (Herba Menthae), *Sān Huáng* (三黄) lotion, *Lú Gān Shí* (炉甘石) lotion or *Fū Kāng Zhǐ Yǎng Shuǐ* (肤康止痒水).

4. SIMPLE PRESCRIPTIONS AND EMPIRICAL FORMULAS

1) *Màn Jīng Zǐ Sǎn* (蔓荆子散)

Grind *Màn jīng zǐ* (Fructus Viticis) 150g into a thin powder. Take 10g per dose. Take with warm wine to treat wind type urticaria.

2) *Chuí Liǔ Tāng* (垂柳汤)

【Ingredients】

垂杨柳	chuí yáng liǔ	500g	Salicaceae

杏仁	xìng rén	150g	Semen Armeniacae Dulcis
白矾	bái fán	100g	Alumen

Decoct the herbs with one and a half deciliters of water until 8 liters remain. Remove the dregs and use the decoction as a wash to treat wind-heat type urticaria.

3) *Shēng Jiàng Sǎn* （升降散）

【Ingredients】

僵蚕	jiāng cán	120g	Bombyx Batryticatus
蝉蜕	chán tuì	60g	Periostracum Cicadae
姜黄	jiāng huáng	180g	Rhizoma Curcumae Longae
大黄	dà huáng	240g	Radix et Rhizoma Rhei

Grind the medicinals into a thin powder and store in a porcelain bottle. Take 6g each time with *huáng jiǔ* (yellow rice wine) 10 ml and *fēng mì* (honey) 15 ml. Drink so as to induce a slight sweat. Avoid the wind for 1-2 days. This treats chronic urticaria.

4) Decoct *chōng wèi zǐ* (Fructus Leonuri), *yún tái* (mutationes), *chán tuì* (Periostracum Cicadae), *cán shā* (Faeces Bombycis), *bái fán* (Alumen) or *líng yáng jiǎo* (Cornu Saigae Tataricae) (burnt to ash) with water or egg whites. Use as an external wash or application.

5) *Sì Chóng Tāng* （四虫汤）

【Ingredients】

乌梢蛇	wū shāo shé	5-10g	Zaocys
广地龙	guǎng dì lóng	9-15g	Pheretima
白僵蚕	bái jiāng cán	6-12g	Bombyx Batryticatu
蝉蜕	chán tuì	3-6g	Periostracum Cicadae

Decoct with water. Take one dose each day to treat chronic urticaria.

6)

面碱	10g	flour alkali
食盐	small amount	table salt
烧酒	100g	strong white wine

Simmer them and apply to itching region. After the wine cools, apply the warm medicine onto affected areas of the skin. This can treat both acute and chronic urticaria.

7) *Yě Qiáng Wēi Gēn* (Rosae Multiflorae Radix) Treatment

Decoct *Yě qiáng wēi gēn* (Rosae Multiflorae Radix) 100g. Take orally each day. One course of treatmen is 7-14 days. This is indicated for stubborn urticaria.

8) *Jiǔ Jiān Ai Yè* （酒煎艾叶）

白酒		100g	white rice wine
生艾叶	shēng ài yè	10g	Folium Artemisiae Argyi

Decoct them until 50g of the decoction remains. Drink the entire decoction in one dose. Take once a day for 3 days.

PROGNOSIS

Acute urticaria has obvious causative factors and a short course of disease. With timely treatment the prognosis is good. Chronic urticaria has complicated causes and a long course of disease, with repeated reoccurrences. Occasionally it can linger for over 10 years. It can be difficult to cure.

PREVENTIVE HEALTHCARE

Because urticaria is an allergic-response type of skin disease, one should avoid contact with allergic substances. Diet regulation and strengthening the body's resistance to diseases should also be part of the treatment. Therefore, in daily life, the following points should be addressed.

Lifestyle Modification

1) Avoid contact with various causative factors.

They include chemical stimulants, inhaled substances (pollen, house dust, animal dander, gasoline, paint, insecticide sprays, and pesticides).

2) Change clothing along with environmental change.

For cases induced by cold and heat, one should try to gradually increase the body's ability to adapt to temperature change.

3) Parasitic infections should be treated by killing the parasites.

In cases of allergic reactions to drugs, the use of drug should be avoided as much as possible. If the drugs can not be avoided, it is advisable to combine them with antihistamines.

4) Pay attention to hygiene and avoid insect bites.

Dietary Recommendation

In terms of diet, avoid spicy foods and alcohol. Dietary regulation is especially important for patients with a history of allergic reactions to certain foods. Commonly reactive foods include protein such as fish, shrimp, crab, beef, and milk, mushrooms, bamboo shoots and seafood. In the allergic patient, these foods are prohibited.

Dietary therapy for urticaria should focus mainly on expelling wind, nourishing and moving blood, and tonifying the Lung and Kidney.

The following are herbs and foods that can be used therapeutically in the diet.

菊花	jú huā	Flos Chrysanthemi
赤芍	chì sháo	Radix Paeoniae Rubra
红花	hóng huā	Flos Carthami

苏叶	sū yè	Folium Perillae
乌梅	wū méi	Fructus Mume
山楂	shān zhā	Fructus Crataegi
木瓜	mù guā	Fructus Chaenomelis
党参	dǎng shēn	Radix Codonopsis
黄芪	huáng qí	Radix Astragali
当归	dāng guī	Radix Angelicae Sinensis
茯苓	fú líng	Poria
山药	shān yào	Rhizoma Dioscoreae
莲子	lián zǐ	Semen Nelumbinis
冬虫夏草	dōng chóng xià cǎo	Cordyceps
蛤蚧	gé jiè	Gecko
糯米		sticky rice
猪胰		pig's pancreas
蜂蜜		honey
元鱼		soft-shelled turtle
竹丝鸡		Zhu si chicken
鹌鹑		quail
羊肉		mutton

1) *Hóng Zǎo Zhū Yí Tāng*（红枣猪胰汤）

红枣	hóng zǎo	250g	Fructus Jujubae
猪胰		1piece	pig's pancrea
食盐		appropriate amount	salt

Simmer them then drink the soup, and eat the dates and pig's pancreas. Treatment is 1 time per day, over two months. This is indicated for a pattern of qi and blood deficiency urticaria.

2) *Hóng Huā Wū Méi Jiǔ*（红花乌梅酒）

红花	hóng huā	100g	Flos Carthami
乌梅	wū méi	100g	Fructus Mume
山楂	shān zhā	100g	Fructus Crataegi
糯米酒		500g	glutinous rice wine

Soak them in 500g of wine made from sticky rice for a week. Then discard the dregs and store the herbal wine in a bottle. Mix 10 ml of the herbal wine with 10 ml water and brown sugar. Drink 2-3 times a day. One course of treatment is 2 weeks. This is indicated for a blood stagnating in the collaterals type of urticaria.

3) *Shēng Dì Yuán Yú Tāng* （生地元鱼汤）

生地	*shēng dì*	18g	Radix Rehmanniae Recens
元鱼		1	soft-shelled turtle
水		200ml	water

Simmer them, once it is cooked, add 10g *sū yè* (Folium Perillae) for a short while. Eat the soup and soft-shelled turtle once every day. One course of treatment is 7 days. This is indicated for a yin deficiency causing exuberant fire pattern type of urticaria.

4) *Dōng Guā Pí Huáng Jú Huā Yǐn* （冬瓜皮黄菊花饮）

冬瓜皮	*dōng guā pí*	20g	Exocarpium Benincasae
黄菊花	*huáng jú huā*	15g	Flos Chrysanthemi
赤芍	*chì sháo*	12g	Radix Paeoniae Rubra

Decoct with an appropriate amount of water for 20-30 minutes.

Discard the dregs and mix the tea with honey. Drink the tea once every day. One course of treatment is 7 days. This is indicated for a wind-heat attacking the exterior type of urticaria.

5) *Mǎ Chǐ Xiàn Zhōu* （马齿苋粥）

马齿苋	*mǎ chǐ xiàn*	60g	Herba Portulacae(minced)
粳米	*jīng mǐ*	50-100g	Oryza satica L.(rice)
红糖		appropriate amount	brown sugar

Cook the herb and rice until they are about eighty percent cooked. Then add an appropriate amount of brown sugar and cook it all together until the rice is soft and cooked. Eat it warm for breakfast and supper.

One course of treatment is 7 days. This is indicated for a blood-heat obstruction pattern of urticaria.

6) *Cù Mù Guā Shēng Jiāng* （醋木瓜生姜）

米醋	mǐ cù	100ml	Vinegar
木瓜	mù guā	60g	Fructus Chaenomelis
生姜	shēng jiāng	9g	Rhizoma Zingiberis Recens

Cook them together in a clay pot until the vinegar is dried. Eat the *mù guā* (Fructus Chaenomelis) and *shēng jiāng* (Rhizoma Zingiberis Recens). This is indicated for a wind-cold attacking the exterior pattern of urticaria.

7) *Dōng Chóng Xià Cǎo Dùn Jī* （冬虫夏草炖鸡）

冬虫夏草	dōng chóng xià cǎo	5g	Cordyceps
枸杞子	gǒu qǐ zǐ	9g	Fructus Lycii
生姜	shēng jiāng	3pieces	Rhizoma Zingiberis Recens
蜜枣	mì zǎo	1	Fructus Jujubae processed with honey
竹丝鸡		half	Zhu si chicken
盐		appropriate amount	salt

Decoct them over a slow fire for 2 hours. Eat the soup and the chicken. This is indicated for a Lung and Kidney deficiency pattern of urticaria.

Regulation of Emotional and Mental Health

Urticaria patients should try to avoid mental irritations and over-exertion. Both mental irritations and fatigue can lead to repeated relapses of the disease. Friends and family members should try to enliven patients so as to prevent patients from becoming depressed. Patients should also try to cultivate a positive and optimistic outlook, and strike a healthy balance between work and rest.

CLINICAL EXPERIENCE OF RENOWNED PHYSICIANS

Empirical Formulas

1) Using *Yǎng Yīn Sōu Fēng Tāng* （养阴搜风汤） to treat internal heat due to yin deficiency and blood dryness causing wind. (Li Shou-shan)

【Ingredients】

何首乌	hé shǒu wū	5-25g	Radix Polygoni Multiflori
全当归	quán dāng guī	10-15g	Radix Angelicae Sinensis
黄芪	huáng qí	20g	Radix Astragali
党参	dǎng shēn	15g	Radix Codonopsi
白鲜皮	bái xiān pí	10-15g	Cortex Dictamni
粉丹皮	fěn dān pí	10-15g	Cortex Moutan
白薇	bái wēi	10-15g	Radix et Rhizoma Cynanchi Atrati
蚕砂	cán shā	15-30g	Faeces Bombycis
乌蛇肉	wū shé ròu	10-15g	Zaocys
白僵蚕	bái jiāng cán	10-15g	Bombyx Batryticatus

【Indications】 There are skin rashes in patches that are smooth and either pale red or the color of the skin. There is also lingering pruritus, repeated reoccurrences, and a prolonged manifestation without cure. The rash is aggravated in the afternoon or at night. It can be caused or aggravated by over-exertion. It can be accompanied by vexation, poor sleep with many dreams, hot sensations in the palms and soles, dry mouth with no desire for drinks, intolerance of cold and heat, a slight red tongue with little moisture, and a deep, thready and wiry pulse.

【Formula Analysis】 *Hé shǒu wū* (Radix Polygoni Multiflori) and *quán dāng guī* (Radix Angelicae Sinensis) nourish yin, tonify blood and moisten dryness to work as the chief herbs. In addition, *hé shǒu wū* (Radix Polygoni Multiflori) has the function of resolving toxins and *quán dāng guī* (Radix Angelicae Sinensis) moves blood. *Bái xiān pí* (Cortex Dictamni) and *fěn dān pí* (Cortex Moutan) clear heat and dispel evils. In addition, *bái xiān pí* (Cortex Dictamni) can dry dampness to resolve toxin, and *fěn dān pí* (Cortex Moutan) can cool the blood to remove blood stasis. The combination of these two herbs can clear dry-heat in blood without causing stagnation. *Bái wēi* (Radix et Rhizoma Cynanchi Atrati) and *cán shā* (Faeces Bombycis) can clear heat and resolve toxin. *Bái wēi* (Radix et Rhizoma Cynanchi Atrati) can enter the blood aspect to disperse swollen abscesses and fire-toxin. *Cán shā* (Faeces Bombycis) moves qi and drains turbid dampness to treat wind-bi type urticaria. The combination of these two herbs can clear heat, drain dampness and expel wind to dispel evil. *Wū shé ròu* (Zaocys) and *bái jiāng cán* (Bombyx Batryticatus) are good at tracking down and removing latent wind in the blood. The combination of these two herbs can strengthen the functions of dispelling wind and relieving itching. This prescription has the function of nourishing yin, tonifying blood and moistening dryness in order to strengthen the right *qi*, clearing heat, removing blood stasis and tracking down latent wind in order to dispel evil. This is an effective prescription for stubborn urticaria.

【Modifications】

For exterior deficiency aggravated by wind, add *huáng qí* (Radix Astragali) and *fáng fēng* (Radix Saposhnikoviae).

For qi deficiency with over-exertion, add *huáng qí* (Radix Astragali).

For yang deficiency aggravated by coldness, add *xiān líng pí* (Epimedium brevicornum Maxim) and *guì zhī* (Ramulus Cinnamomi).

For severe pruritus, add *quán xiē* (Scorpio) and *chán yī* (Periostracum Cicadae).

For extreme pruritus, use *bǎi bù jiǔ* (*bǎi bù* [Radix Stemonae] 100g, soaked for 3 days and nights in 500 ml of strong alcohol) as an external application.

(Shan Shu-jian, Chen Zi-hua: Editors-in-chief. *Clinical Case Recordings of Modern Famous Chinese Medicine Doctors-the Category of Surgery* 当代名医鉴证金鉴 . 外科卷 . Chinese Medicinal Publishing House, 1999： 195.)

2) *Gù Wèi Yù Fēng Tāng* （固卫御风汤）to treat cold urticaria (Zhu Ren-kang)

【Ingredients】

炙黄芪	zhì huáng qí	9g	Radix Astragali（processed）
防风	fáng fēng	9g	Radix Saposhnikoviae
炒白术	chǎo bái zhú	9g	Rhizoma Atractylodis Macrocephalae（stir-fried）
桂技	guì zhī	9g	Ramulus Cinnamomi
赤芍	chì sháo	9g	Radix Paeoniae Rubra
白芍	bái sháo	9g	Radix Paeoniae Alba
生姜	shēng jiāng	3pieces	Rhizoma Zingiberis Recens
大枣	dà zǎo	7	Fructus Jujubae

【Indications】 This treats urticaria that lingers for several years and appears occasionally. On very cold days, the urticaria can be caused by cold wind. Then there is severe pruritus, and wheals that can occur on the exposed parts of the body, such as the head, face, hands and feet. The wheals remain until the warm spring, when they disappear on their own. They can be accompanied by a pale complexion, cold limbs, aversion to cold, numbness of the hands and feet, vertigo and dizziness, a pale tongue body with a thin white coat, and a soggy and thready pulse.

【Formula Analysis】 This formula is *Yù Píng Fēng Sǎn* with *Guì Zhī Tāng* (桂枝汤). *Huáng qí* (Radix Astragali), *bái zhú* (Rhizoma Atractylodis Macrocephalae) and *fáng fēng* (Radix Saposhnikoviae) consolidate the exterior and protect the body from wind. *Guì zhī* (Ramulus Cinnamomi), *bái sháo* (Radix Paeoniae Alba), *shēng jiāng* (Rhizoma Zingiberis Recens) and *dà zǎo* (Fructus Jujubae) regulate the *ying* and the *wei*, and expel wind-cold. They are assisted by *chì sháo* (Radix Paeoniae Alba) to move the blood and dispel wind. *Wū méi* (Fructus Mume), and *wǔ wèi zǐ* (Fructus

Schisandrae Chinensis) have a sour flavor and an astringent property, and are used for a lingering course of disease.

(Guang An Men Hospital of Chinese Medicine Research Institute. *Clinical Experience Recordings of Zhu Ren-kang- the Category of Dermal Surgery* 朱仁康临床经验集·皮肤外科. The people's Medical Publishing House, 1979：236.)

3) *Wū Shé Chán Yī Tāng* （乌蛇蝉衣汤）to treat wind-heat attacking the exterior type of urticaria (Zhang Xi-jun)

【Ingredients】

乌蛇	wū shé	10g	Zaocys
蝉衣	chán yī	6g	Periostracum Cicadae
赤芍	chì sháo	9g	Radix Paeoniae Rubra
防风	fáng fēng	6g	Radix Saposhnikoviae
荆芥	jīng jiè	6g	Herba Schizonepetae
薄荷	bò hé	6g	Herba Menthae
千里光	qiān lǐ guāng	30g	Senecio vulgaris
虎耳草	hǔ ěr cǎo	30g	Saxifraga stolonifera
白鲜皮	bái xiān pí	6g	Cortex Dictamni

【Indications】 This treats red wheals that are spread over the whole body. They disappear and reappear on their own, and are aggravated in the morning and at night. The wheals are accompanied by disturbed sleep, a red tongue body with a thin white coat, and a slippery and rapid pulse.

(Shi Yu-guang, Shan Shu-jian. Editors-in-Chief: *Essentials Of Modern Chineses Medicine Doctors' Clinic: Dermatology* 当代名医临证精华. 皮肤病专辑. Ancient Books Of Chinese Medicine Publishing Office, 1991：18）

Selected Case Studies

(1) Zhou Feng-wu's Case Studies —Urticaria Due to Heat Toxin

Mr. Yang, 45 years old, male purchasing agent.

【Initial Visit】 August 26th 1969. Due to furuncles on the external auditory canal, this patient received penicillin injections for over a month, that cured him of the swelling. Subsequently, the patient had a latent rash over his entire body. This rash had lumps that were burning red and swollen, extremely itchy and difficult to endure. The diagnosis was urticaria. He had been treated with Chinese medicine without effect. Moreover, the purpura and pruritus were aggravated over the whole body. In the evening at 10 o'clock, the patient's body was covered with a thick quilt. Then he sat near the edge of the bed and suddenly removed the quilt and got up from the bed. He was fidgety, with mental-emotional vexation and agitation. He was groaning endlessly. He had chills and a feverish sensation over his body. The burning sensation could be felt by touch. His skin was swollen, and the rashes had coagulated into patches on the head and face. There was erythema, purpura and black spots that spread over the four limbs and back. This was accompanied by indescribably severe pruritus. Because of incautious hot-pack applications, there were exudating blisters on both wrists. He had a poor appetite, and thirst with desire for drinks (up to 5 bottles of water a day). He had no bowel movements for 2 days, and scanty and red urine as if it was obstructed. His pulse was rapid, racing, long and large. There was a thick tongue coat all over the tongue, with yellow-dryness in the center.

【Pattern Differentiation】 External attack by wind evil with latent summer-heat internally, extreme heat in the *Yangming* meridian, causing a pestilent maculae pattern.

【Treatment Principle】 Clear *Yangming* pathogenic heat, induce eruptions to expel toxins.

【Prescription】

| 生石膏（先煎） | shēng shí gāo | 60g | Gypsum Fibrosum (unprocessed) (decoct first) |
| 肥知母 | féi zhī mǔ | 12g | Rhizoma Anemarrhenae |

大玄参	dà xuán shēn	15g	Radix Scrophulariae
忍冬藤	rěn dōng téng	15g	Caulis Lonicerae Japonicae
金银花	jīn yín huā	15g	Flos Lonicerae Japonicae
蒲公英	pú gōng yīng	15g	Herba Taraxaci
飞滑石	fēi huá shí	15g	Talcum（prepared from elutriation）
生大黄（后入）	shēng dà huáng	9g	Radix et Rhizoma Rhei (decoct later)
淡竹叶	dàn zhú yè	9g	Herba Lophatheri
生甘草	shēng gān cǎo	6g	Radix et Rhizoma Glycyrrhizae
粳米	jīng mǐ	15g	rice

Decoct in water. Take warm, twice.

【Second Visit】 August 29th. There was no improvement after the treatment. He had severe pruritus over the whole body, leading to an inability to fall asleep at night. He also had thirst with fever, irritability, restlessness, a rapid and racing pulse, and a thick-white tongue coat spread over the entire tongue. The yellow coat had disappeared. According to the disease condition, relieving itching is the first goal. The patient was asked to eat more watermelon, or use the watermelon as a drink. The patient was treated with the following internal and external prescriptions:

Prescription for oral administration:

白鲜皮	bái xiān pí	12g	Cortex Dictamni
净蝉蜕	jìng chán tuì	9g	Periostracum Cicadae
地肤子	dì fū zǐ	12g	Fructus Kochiae
海桐皮	hǎi tóng pí	12g	Cortex Erythrinae
南薄荷	nán bò hé	6g	Herba Menthae
荆芥穗	jīng jiè suì	6g	Spica Schizonepetae
青防风	qīng fáng fēng	6g	Radix Saposhnikoviae
银花	yín huā	18g	Flos Lonicerae Japonicae
赤芍药	chì sháo yào	9g	Radix Paeoniae Rubra
生大黄（后入）	shēng dà huáng	9g	Radix et Rhizoma Rhei (unprocessed) (decoct later)
生甘草	shēng gān cǎo	6g	Radix et Rhizoma Glycyrrhizae

Decoct with water, take twice.

Prescription for external use:

生大黄	shēng dà huáng	60g	Radix et Rhizoma Rhei (unprocessed)
香白芷	xiāng bái zhǐ	30g	Radix Angelicae Dahuricae
青黛	qīng dài	15g	Indigo Naturalis

The three kinds of herbs were ground into a thin powder and mixed with tea for external application on the skin lesion or the itching areas. Use 3 or 4 times a day.

【Third Visit】 August 30th. The patient combined the internal and external treatments with eating 5 kilograms of watermelon. The pruritus was relieved a little but he still had fever, thirst, and dark–brown stool, 3-4 times a day, like soy sauce. The skin rashes on the wrists and legs subsidized gradually but reoccurred on the chest. He had an obstructive sensation in the throat, 4 hours of sleep at night, and a large pulse. The white coat disappeared from the tip of the tongue and was replaced by a slightly thinner coat in the center and root. Heat toxin has the tendency to be dispelled and discharged downward and should be treated by the method of clearing heat and resolving toxin.

【Prescription】

生石膏	shēng shí gāo	45g	Gypsum Fibrosum (unprocessed)
肥知母	féi zhī mǔ	12g	Rhizoma Anemarrhenae
大玄参	dà xuán shēn	12g	Radix Scrophulariae
苦桔梗	kǔ jié gěng	9g	Radix Platycodonis
牛蒡子	niú bàng zǐ	9g	Fructus Arctii
射干片	shè gān piàn	6g	Rhizoma Belamcandae (cut into slices)
南薄荷	nán bò hé	6g	Herba Menthae
金银花	jīn yín huā	15g	Flos Lonicerae Japonicae
净蝉蜕	jìng chán tuì	9g	Periostracum Cicadae
白鲜皮	bái xiān pí	12g	Cortex Dictamni
飞滑石	fēi huá shí	12g	Talcum（prepared from elutriation）

| 淡黄芩 | dàn huáng qín | 9g | Radix Scutellariae |
| 生甘草 | shēng gān cǎo | 6g | Radix et Rhizoma Glycyrrhizae (unprocessed) |

Decoct in water . Take warm, twice.

【Fourth Visit】 August 31st. The skin lesions disappeared from the legs, arms and back but not completely from the head, face or chest. He had a good appetite, thirst with desire for cold drinks, an aversion to cold, fever, stool in the color of soy sauce, and excessive yellow urine. His pulse was rapid, and the slightly thin coat had disappeared from the root of his tongue. He was asked to eat watermelon continuously. The treatment principle from the last treatment was used, with some modifications to the original prescription.

【Prescription】

生石膏	shēng shí gāo	45g	Gypsum Fibrosum (unprocessed)
肥知母	féi zhī mǔ	12g	Rhizoma Anemarrhenae
大玄参	dà xuán shēn	15g	Radix Scrophulariae
南薄荷	nán bò hé	6g	Herba Menthae
金银花	jīn yín huā	15g	Flos Lonicerae Japonicae
忍冬藤	rěn dōng téng	15g	Caulis Lonicerae Japonicae
淡黄芩	dàn huáng qín	9g	Radix Scutellariae
净蝉蜕	jìng chán tuì	9g	Periostracum Cicadae
淡竹叶	dàn zhú yè	9g	Herba Lophatheri
荆芥穗	jīng jiè suì	4.5g	Spica Schizonepetae
白鲜皮	bái xiān pí	12g	Cortex Dictamni
大青皮	dà qīng pí	9g	Pericarpium Citri Reticulatae Viride
生甘草	shēng gān cǎo	4.5g	Radix et Rhizoma Glycyrrhizae

Decoct in water. Take warm, twice.

【Fifth Visit】 September 2nd. The skin rashes disappeared completely but he still had pruritus. He had a good appetite, thirst with a desire for cold drinks, fever on the lower body, and the stool, 3-4 times a day, became red. He had a rapid pulse, and a greasy-white coat. It was treated by the method of clearing summer-heat and dampness.

【Prescription】

生石膏	shēng shí gāo	30g	Gypsum Fibrosum (unprocessed)
肥知母	féi zhī mǔ	12g	Rhizoma Anemarrhenae
金石斛	jīn shí hú	12g	Caulis Dendrobii
青竹茹	qīng zhú rú	9g	Caulis Bambusae in Taenia
扁豆花	biǎn dòu huā	15g	Semen Lablab Album
金银花	jīn yín huā	18g	Flos Lonicerae Japonicae
淡黄芩	dàn huáng qín	9g	Radix Scutellariae
生黄柏	shēng huáng bǎi	3g	Cortex Phellodendri Amurensis (unprocessed)
飞滑石	fēi huá shí	15g	Talcum（prepared from elutriation）
南薄荷	nán bò hé	6g	Herba Menthae
白鲜皮	bái xiān pí	9g	Cortex Dictamni
地肤子	dì fū zǐ	9g	Fructus Kochiae
生甘草	shēng gān cǎo	3g	Radix et Rhizoma Glycyrrhizae

Decoct in water .Take warm, twice.

【Sixth Visit】 September 4th. His skin rashes disappeared completely, and the desire for cold drinks was lessened. He had a slight fever and pruritus. He had a slightly rapid pulse, a thin-white tongue coat, and yellow stool. The former prescription was modified by adding *běi shā shēn* (Radix Glehniae), *mài dōng* (Radix Ophiopogonis), *qīng hāo* (Herba Artemisiae Annuae) and *bái wēi* (Radix et Rhizoma Cynanchi Atrati), and by discarding *jiǎn huáng qín* (Radix Scutellariae), *huáng bǎi* (Cortex Phellodendri Chinensis), *huá shí* (Talcum), and *zhú rú* (Caulis Bambusae in Taenia). After 4 dosages, this patient was cured and had a good appetite. He was told to eat less food at each meal, and to eat more meals in a day. This would prevent reoccurrences from improper diet.

(Dong Jian-hua: Editor-in-chief. *Essentials of Modern Famous Chineses Medicine Doctors' Clinical Cases* 中国现代名中医医案精华 . Beijing Publishing Press, 1990.93）

(2) Zhu Ren-kang's Case Studies—Qi Deficient and Not Consolidated.

Mr. Zhang, 69 year old, male.

【Initial Visit】 November 3rd 1972. The patient suffered from repeated urticaria with sneezing for 5 years. Each time it lasted for about 10 days. This July after eating beans and peaches the skin rashes reoccurred and lasted for 4 months. There was no successful treatment effect. Physical examination: Diffuse skin rashes on the whole body in different sizes, coagulated into patches, with white color in the center, a pale tongue body with a normal coat, and a thready and slippery pulse.

【Pattern Differentiation】 Lung qi deficiency, with *wei* and exterior not consolidated, and external wind easily attacking.

【Treatment Principle】 Tonify the Lung and consolidate the exterior in order to protect the body from external wind evil.

【Prescription】

黄芪	huáng qí	9g	Radix Astragali
沙参	shā shēn	9g	Radix Glehniae
防风	fáng fēng	9g	Radix Saposhnikoviae
柴胡	chái hú	6g	Radix Bupleuri
陈皮	chén pí	6g	Pericarpium Citri Reticulatae
茯苓皮	fú líng pí	9g	Poria (skin)
地肤子	dì fū zǐ	9g	Fructus Kochiae
白鲜皮	bái xiān pí	9g	Cortex Dictamni
大枣	dà zǎo	5	Fructus Jujubae

After five dosages there was no reoccurrence.

【Second Visit】 September 4th, 1973. No reoccurrence after treatment last year. This July after contracting a common cold, the urticaria reoccurred without being cured until now. It can be controlled slightly with anti-allergic inhalers, but there is still some reoccurrence. The pulse was wiry and slippery, and the tongue body was red with a normal coat

【Pattern Differentiation】 Lung losing their clearing and depurating, and the exterior contracting wind.

【Treatment Principle】 Consolidate the exterior and protect body from wind evil, keep the Lung *qi* pure and descendant.

【Prescription】

沙参	shā shēn	9g	Radix Glehniae
防风	fáng fēng	6g	Radix Saposhnikoviae
辛荑花	xīn yí huā	3g	Flos Magnoliae
黄芪	huáng qí	9g	Radix Astragali
炒白术	chǎo bái zhú	9g	Rhizoma Atractylodis Macrocephalae (stir-fried)
桑白皮	sāng bái pí	6g	Cortex Mori
枇杷叶	pí pa yè	9g	Folium Eriobotryae
甘草	gān cǎo	6g	Radix et Rhizoma Glycyrrhizae
大枣	dà zǎo	5	Fructus Jujubae

【Third Visit】 September 10th. After taking the herbs there were less wheals, and a decrease in the sneezing and runny nose. The tongue coat and pulse were the same as last time. The previous prescription, with modifications, was used. Discard *pí pa yè* (Folium Eriobotryae) and *sāng bái pí* (Cortex Mori), add *wǔ wèi zǐ* (Fructus Schisandrae Chinensis) 9g and *chái hú* (Radix Bupleuri) 6g. It was decoct in water, and taken for five doses.

【Fourth Visit】 September 15th. All the symptoms disappeared except for a slight cough. The *chái hú* (Radix Bupleuri) was discarded and *qián hú* (Radix Peucedani) 9g was added.

【Fifth Visit】 September 22nd. All the symptoms were relieved except for cough. He had a normal tongue coat and strong pulse in the cun position. The *xīn yí huā* (Flos Magnoliae) was discarded, and *jié gěng* (Radix Platycodonis) 9g, *bǎi hé* (Bulbus Lilii) 9g and *niú bàng zǐ* (Fructus Arctii) 9g were added in order to descend the Lung *qi*. After 5 dosages, the patient was cured.

(Guang An Men Hospital of Chinese Medicine Researching Institute edit. *Clinical Experience' Recordings of Zhu Ren-kang- the Category of Dermal Surgery* 朱仁康经验集 . 皮肤外科 .The People's Medical Publishing House, 1979：112.)

(3) Zhao Bing-nan's Case Studies —Mixture of Wind-Cold & Damp-Heat

Ms Li, 41 year old, female.

【Initial Visit】 February 10th, 1971. For 10 years she had continuous red lumps on the whole body, occurring mainly on the trunk and four limbs, and accompanied by severe pruritus. The condition was relieved and aggravated spontaneously. The skin rashes were aggravated in the morning and at night, especially in the winter after going to bed at night. Even in summer it didn't disappear. The rash was treated without effect. Physical examination: Diffused flat light red apophysis in the size of finger nails or coins, coagulating into big patches with different shapes spreading on the four limbs. She had a pale tongue body with a white coat, and a deep and moderate pulse. It was diagnosed as chronic urticaria.

【Pattern Differentiation】 Accumulation of dampness with wind-cold evil transforming into heat, with lingering wind-cold and damp-heat manifesting on the skin.

【Treatment Principle】 Harmonize yin, yang, qi and blood. Also clear heat, and dispel coldness, calm wind, and resolve dampness.

【Prescription】

五加皮	wǔ jiā pí	9g	Cortex Acanthopanacis
桑白皮	sāng bái pí	9g	Cortex Mori
地骨皮	dì gǔ pí	9g	Cortex Lycii
丹皮	dān pí	9g	Cortex Moutan
干姜	gān jiāng	9g	Rhizoma Zingiberis
陈皮	chén pí	9g	Pericarpium Citri Reticulatae

扁豆皮	biǎn dòu pí	9g	Semen Lablab Album (skin)
茯苓皮	fú líng pí	9g	Poria (skin)
白鲜皮	bái xiān pí	9g	Cortex Dictamni
陈皮	chén pí	9g	Pericarpium Citri Reticulatae
大腹皮	dà fù pí	9g	Pericarpium Arecae
当归	dāng guī	9g	Radix Angelicae Sinensis
浮萍	fú píng	9g	Herba Spirodelae

【Second Visit】 February 17th. After 7 doses of the prescription, the skin rashes markedly decreased. There were a few skin rashes in the morning when the patient went out and no skin rashes at night.

【Third Visit】 February 26th. After taking another 4 doses, the skin rashes didn't reoccur. This patient was clinically cured after 3 more doses.

(Shi Yu-guang, Shan Shu-jian. Editors-in-chief. *Essentials Of Modern Chinese Medicine Doctors' Clinic: Dermatosis* 当代名医临证精华·皮肤病专辑 . Ancient Books of Chinese Medicine Publishing Office, 1992.89.)

(4) He Ru-han's Case Studies —Dampness Stagnation in the Middle Jiao, External Contraction of Wind Evil

Ms Cao, 20 year old, female.

【Initial Visit】 May 27th, 1980

The patient had flushed skin over the whole body, along with swollen lumps and pruritus. This had lasted for over 20 days, and was aggravated by heat. She was treated in a hospital with oral medicine and calcium gluconate injections. Her skin rashes occasionally disappeared and reoccurred. The patient had abdominal distension, but a normal appetite without stool for 2 days. Her tongue body was red with a yellow-greasy coat, and her pulse was wiry, slippery and rapid on both sides. The physical examination revealed a yellowish complexion, and flat, edematous, light red urticaria spread over the four limbs. The wheals were different sizes and some of them looked like patches, accompanied by obvious scratch marks.

【Pattern Differentiation】 Irregular diet, damp stagnation in the Middle Jiao, loose interstitial spaces, externally contracted wind evil.

【Treatment Principle】 Dispel wind and clear hear, assist to promote digestion so as to relieve food stagnation.

【Prescription】

金银花	jīn yín huā	12g	Flos Lonicerae Japonicae
白鲜皮	bái xiān pí	10g	Cortex Dictamni
黄菊花	huáng jú huā	6g	Flos Chrysanthem
地肤子	dì fū zǐ	10g	Fructus Kochia
茯苓皮	fú líng pí	10g	Poria (skin)
防风	fáng fēng	6g	Radix Saposhnikoviae
荆芥穗	jīng jiè suì	6g	Spica Schizonepetae
赤芍药	chì sháo yào	10g	Radix Paeoniae Rubra
枳实	zhǐ shí	4.5g	Fructus Aurantii Immaturus
厚朴	hòu pò	6g	Cortex Magnoliae Officinalis
大黄	dà huáng	10g	Radix et Rhizoma Rhei

External use: *Bai Bu Jiu* 100 ml mixed with *Zhi Yang Yao Feng* 3g.

【Second Visit】 After 2 doses of the prescription, the old skin rashes were relieved and there was a decrease in new skin rashes. There was also less pruritus, open bowels, slightly relieved abdominal distention, and yellow urine. The tongue and pulse manifestation was the same as the previous visit. The former prescription was modified as follows. Use *jīn yín téng* (Lonicera japonica Thunb) 12g to take place of *jīn yín huā* (Flos Lonicerae Japonicae), reduce *dà huáng* (Radix et Rhizoma Rhei) to 6g. The external used prescription remained the same.

【Third Visit】 After another 2 doses the skin rashes disappeared, though occasionally there were 1 to 2 skin lesions and slight pruritus. She had a poor appetite and sluggish bowel movements. The patient's tongue coat was thin-yellow, and the pulse was wiry and slippery. A new formula was prescribed based on the previous prescription. Methods to clear heat and transform stagnated heat were also used.

【Prescription】

金银藤	jīn yín téng	12g	Lonicera japonica Thunb
白鲜皮	bái xiān pí	10g	Cortex Dictamni
黄菊花	huáng jú huā	10g	Flos Chrysanthem
焦建曲	jiāo jiàn qū	10g	Massa Medicata Fermentata (charred)
茯苓皮	fú líng pí	10g	Poria (skin)
赤芍药	chì sháo yào	10g	Radix Paeoniae Rubra
焦山楂	jiāo shān zhā	10g	Fructus Crataegi (charred)
橘皮	jú pí	6g	Exocarpium Citri Rubrum
竹茹	zhú rú	6g	Caulis Bambusae in Taenia

After 3 dosages there were no reoccurrences and the patient was cured.

（Beijing Chinese Medicine Hospital, Capital Associated University Chinese Medicine College Editor-in-chief. *Comprehensive Recording of Clinical Experience of Famous Chinese Medicine Doctors (second half of the book)* 名老中医经验全编（下）. Beijing Publishing House, 1994，462~463.）

(5) Xuan Guo-wei's Case Studies —Deficiency of the Lung & Kidney

Ms Zhang, 46 year old, female.

【Initial Visit】 March 18th, 1988

The patient suffered from repeated bouts of skin rashes and pruritus over her whole body for over a year. She had been diagnosed with nephropyelitis and had been cured with treatment. After that she had shortness of breath during activity, soreness and weakness of lower back and knees, and tidal fever with night sweats. Half a year later, after an external contracted fever, she developed that urticaria spread over the whole body, along with slight pruritus. She had repeated reoccurrences even after various kinds of treatment. Physical examination revealed light red and pale skin rashes on the face, neck, chest and back. She had pale lips, a pale tongue body with a scanty coat, and a thready pulse.

【Pattern Differentiation】 Deficiency of the Lung and Kidney.

【Treatment Principle】 Tonify the Lung and constrain the Kidney

【Prescription】

山茱萸	shān zhū yú	15g	Fructus Corni
怀山药	huái shān yào	15g	Rhizoma
茯苓	fú líng	15g	Poria
熟地黄	shú dì huáng	15g	Radix Rehmanniae Praeparata
牡丹皮	mǔ dān pí	15g	Cortex Moutan
泽泻	zé xiè	15g	Rhizoma Alismatis
乌梅	wū méi	15g	Fructus Mume
何首乌	hé shǒu wū	15g	Radix Polygoni Multiflori Praeparata cum Succo Glycines Sotae
刺蒺藜	cì jí lí	15g	Fructus Tribuli
五味子	wǔ wèi zǐ	10g	Fructus Schisandrae Chinensis
甘草	gān cǎo	9g	Radix et Rhizoma Glycyrrhizae

Decoct with water twice, divide one dose into two and drink twice daily. This patient was cured after one and a half months. After one year, there was no reoccurrence.

【Comments】 Chronic urticaria is similar to the "Insidious Rash" *yǐn zhěn* (瘾疹) and "Wind Rash" *fēng zhěn* (风疹) recorded in Chinese literature. This case was caused by deficiency of the Lung and Kidney and was treated by tonifying the Kidney and astringing the Lung. The prescription was a modificated *Liù Wèi Dì Huáng Wán*. *Liù Wèi Dì Huáng Tāng* (六味地黄汤) nourishes yin, tonifes the Kidneys, and strengthens Kidney *yin* to restrict the hyperactivity of Kidney *yang*. *Hé shǒu wū* (Radix Polygoni Multiflori) can enter the Liver and Kidney meridians to tonify deficient *jing* (essence) and blood. *Wǔ wèi zǐ* (Fructus Schisandrae Chinensis) and *wū méi* (Fructus Mume) can astringe the Lung and

Kidney. *Cì jí lí* (Fructus Tribuli) dispels wind and relieves itching. *Gān cǎo* (Radix et Rhizoma Glycyrrhizae) harmonizes the actions of the other herbs. This prescription is used to treat chronic urticaria belonging to a Lung and Kidney deficiency pattern.

(Xuan Guo-wei. *Intractable Skin Diseases Treated With Tonifying Kidney* 补肾法治疗疑难皮肤病. New Journal of Traditional Chinese Medicine. 1993，(9)：44)

(6) Lin He-he's Case Studies—Cold Evil Depressing the Exterior, Residual Toxin Internally Smoldering

Ms Zhang, 44 year old, female doctor

【**Initial Visit**】 March 28th, 1981.

In the winter of the past year, the patient contracted measles, and during that time she developed pustules. The patient's condition was perilous, but she got better. However, a few days later she contracted a secondary wind evil in the flesh and skin. On the skin emerged kernel-shaped wheals, along with whole-body pruritus. After scratching they blended together into rings. There was flushing and scorching heat. When she slept covered with a quilt, the burning sensation and pruritus were aggravated. She was unable to sleep in daytime or at night. This lasted for 4 months and was treated with Chinese medicine and biomedicine but without effect, so she came asked for a consultation. The body temperature and blood pressure were normal, and the blood leukocyte classification was E16%. The tongue had a yellow-white and slight greasy coat with fluids, and the pulse was floating, faint and tight. The diagnosis was urticaria.

【**Pattern Differentiation**】 Cold evil depressing the exterior, residual measles toxin smoldering in the interior.

【**Treatment Principle**】 Diffuse and scatter the exterior evil, assist in order to clear, disinhibit, and cool the blood.

【Prescription】

麻黄	má huáng	9g	Caulis Trachelospermi
连翘	lián qiào	9g	Fructus Forsythiae
杏仁	xìng rén	9g	Armeniacae Semen Amarum
赤小豆	chì xiǎo dòu	15g	Semen Phaseoli
生地	shēng dì	9g	Radix Rehmanniae Recens
丹皮	dān pí	9g	Cortex Moutan
防风	fáng fēng	9g	Radix Saposhnikoviae
蝉衣	chán yī	6g	Periostracum Cicadae
生甘草	shēng gān cǎo	3g	Radix et Rhizoma Glycyrrhizae (raw)
生姜	shēng jiāng	6g	Rhizoma Zingiberis Recens
大枣	dà zǎo	7	Fructus Jujubae

It was made into 3 doses. 1/3 of the thickened decoction was used for external application. After one dose, the skin rashes mostly disappeared, with only some diffused rashes remaining on the upper limbs and chest. There was decreased pruritus, and no burning sensation on the skin. Now she can fall asleep covered with a quilt. Her pulse was moderate, and the tongue had a normal coat but no fluids. Discard *má huáng* (Herba Ephedrae), *xìng rén* (Semen Armeniacae Amarum) and *shēng jiāng* (Rhizoma Zingiberis Recens). Add *tài zǐ shēn* (Radix Pseudostellariae) 10g, *shān yào* (Rhizoma Dioscoreae) 10g and *yì mǐ* (Semen Coicis) 10g. After 4 more doses, this patient was cured and had no reoccurrence for several years.

【Comments】 *Má Huáng Lián Qiào Chì Xiǎo Dòu Tāng* (麻黄连翘赤小豆汤) was first recorded in *Discussion of Cold Damage* (伤寒论 , *Shāng Hán Lùn*) 263rd comment. "For cold-damage and stagnated internal heat manifested as jaundice, treat with *Má Huáng Lián Qiào Chì Xiǎo Dòu Tāng* (麻黄连翘赤小豆汤)" To treat internal damp-heat with jaundice, this prescription has the function of releasing the exterior and dispelling evils, clearing and draining toxin. For this case, onset of urticaria in adulthood, toxins are internally retained and cold evil accumulates on the exterior. This damages the *ying* and *wei*, causing a pathogenic change both internally and externally leading to skin rashes with burning sensations and pruritus. *Má huáng* (Herba Ephedrae) and *xìng rén* (Semen Armeniacae Amarum) dispel the external evil, *lián qiào* (Fructus Forsythiae) and *chì xiǎo dòu* (Semen Phaseoli) clear the remaining toxin, *dān pí* (Cortex Moutan) takes place of *zǐ bǎi pí* (Cortex Catalpa ovata G. Don) to treat the burning sensation on the skin, *shēng dì huáng* (Radix Rehmanniae Recens) clears heat and cools the blood, *fáng fēng* (Radix Saposhnikoviae) and *chán yī* (Periostracum Cicadae) are important herbs to track wind and relieve itching, *shēng jiāng* (Rhizoma Zingiberis Recens) assists *má huáng* (Herba Ephedrae) to dispel the exterior evil, *dà zǎo* (Fructus Jujubae) helps nourish yin, and *shēng gān cǎo* (Radix et Rhizoma Glycyrrhizae) harmonizes the actions of the other herbs. The key point in treating this stubborn urticaria of 4 months is a good understanding of the pathogenesis. The pathogenesis derives from lingering toxins and should be treated by the combination of internal and external therapies.

(Shi Yu-guang, Shan Shu-jian. Editors-in-chief. *Essentials Of Modern Chinese Medicine Doctors' Clinic: Dermatosis* 当代名医临证精华 · 皮肤病专辑. Ancient Books of Chinese Medicine Publishing Office, 1992.106.)

Discussions

1. Zhu Ren-kang's five patterns of differentiation and treatment of urticaria.

Zhu Ren-kang believes that urticaria is caused by internal factors, external factors or the combination of both internal and external factors. During the acute stage, it can be divided into wind-heat and wind-dampness patterns and should be treated by the method of coursing wind and clearing heat, or dispelling wind and draining dampness. Chronic urticaria is stubborn and difficult to cure. Effective treatments should be based on pattern differentiation and cause. If wind evil is depressed for a long time without being dispelled, use large doses of herbs that have the function of tracking wind to dispel evil. Also, in the cases of *wei qi* not consolidated with wind and cold exposure, it is suitable to treat by the method consolidating the *wei* so as to resist wind. For cases that have an internal etiology at the same time as an exterior etiology (such as wind evil attacking the exterior along with an improper diet, and failure of transportation due to Spleen deficiency), the symptoms can include stomach pain, vomiting, abdominal pain, and diarrhea. This pattern should be treated by the method of warming the Middle Jiao, strengthening the Spleen, regulating qi flow and stopping pain. In addition, there are other common internal etiologies, including blood-heat and blood-stagnation producing wind. Burning sensations, stabbing itching, and demographic scratch marks are very common and can be caused by internal wind induced by external wind. In those cases, the disease should be treated by the method of cooling blood and clearing heat in order to extinguish internal wind. In a blood stagnation pattern, blood stagnates in the meridians and interstitial spaces, and this gives rise to a disharmony between the *ying* and *wei*. When this occurs, urticaria can arise. This should be treated by strongly moving blood and dispelling wind. "To treat wind, first treat the blood; when blood moves then wind is spontaneously extinguished." (治风先治血，血行风自灭。) Cases of mixed cold and heat patterns should treat both the cold and heat aspects. In conclusion, because of the complicated etiologies, effective treatments should be based on pattern differentiation.

(1) Wind-heat pattern

Generally speaking, this is mainly seen in cases of acute urticaria, but it can still be a part of chronic urticaria. Because of external attack by wind-heat, there can be symptoms including patchy red skin lesions, lingering pain, and pruritus. In severe cases, there can be swelling of the face and lips. Skin rashes can be easily brought out by sweating and fever. There can be a dry pharynx and vexation. The tongue is red, with a thin white or thin yellow coat. The pulse is wiry, slippery and rapid.

【Treatment Principle】 Course wind, clear heat, assisted by cooling blood.

【Prescription】 *Xiāo Fēng Qīng Rè Yǐn* (消风清热饮)

【Ingredients】

荆芥	jīng jiè	9g	Herba Schizonepetae
防风	fáng fēng	9g	Radix Saposhnikoviae
浮萍	fú píng	9g	Herba Spirodelae
蝉衣	chán yī	9g	Periostracum Cicadae
当归	dāng guī	9g	Radix Angelicae Sinensis
赤芍	chì sháo	9g	Radix Paeoniae Rubra
大青叶	dà qīng yè	9g	Folium Isatidis
黄芩	huáng qín	9g	Radix Scutellariae

Or a modified *Shū Fēng Qīng Rè Yǐn* (疏风清热饮)

【Ingredients】

荆芥	jīng jiè	9g	Herba Schizonepetae
防风	fáng fēng	9g	Radix Saposhnikoviae
牛蒡子	niú bàng zǐ	9g	Fructus Arctii
白蒺藜	bái jí lí	9g	Fructus Tribuli
蝉衣	chán yī	9g	Periostracum Cicadae
生地	shēng dì huáng	15g	Radix Rehmanniae Recens
丹参	dān shēn	9g	Radix et Rhizoma Salviae Miltiorrhizae
赤芍	chì sháo	9g	Radix Paeoniae Rubra
炒山栀	chǎo zhī zǐ	9g	Fructus Gardeniae Praeparatus
黄芩	huáng qín	9g	Radix Scutellariae
金银花	jīn yín huā	9g	Flos Lonicerae Japonicae
连翘	lián qiào	9g	Fructus Forsythiae
生甘草	shēng gān cǎo	6g	Radix et Rhizoma Glycyrrhizae

In cases of long-term (1-2 years) depressed wind-heat evil that fails to be dispelled and discharged, there can be symptoms including bright red skin rashes in big patches, and a red tongue body with a yellow coat.

【Treatment Principle】 Track wind and clear heat.

【Prescription】 *Wū Shé Qū Fēng Tāng* (乌蛇驱风汤)

【Ingredients】

乌蛇	wū shé	9g	Zaocys
蝉衣	chán yī	6g	Periostracum Cicadae
荆芥	jīng jiè	9g	Herba Schizonepetae
防风	fáng fēng	9g	Radix Saposhnikoviae
羌活	qiāng huó	9g	Rhizoma et Radix Notopterygii
白芷	bái zhǐ	6g	Radix Angelicae Dahuricae
黄连	huáng lián	9g	Rhizoma Coptidis
黄芩	huáng qín	9g	Radix Scutellariae
金银花	jīn yín huā	9g	Flos Lonicerae Japonicae
连翘	lián qiào	9g	Fructus Forsythiae
甘草	gān cǎo	6g	Radix et Rhizoma Glycyrrhizae

(2) Wind-cold pattern

Because the *wei* and exterior are not consolidated, wind cold externally sneak-attacks, and there is a disharmony between the *ying* and the *wei*. Skin lesions occur on parts of the body that are exposed to wind and cold. It can manifest as light red or pale skin rashes. There can also be a pale tongue body with a thin white coat, and a tight or moderate pulse.

【Treatment Principle】 Consolidate the *wei* and harmonize the *ying*

【Prescription】 Modified *Gù Wèi Yù Fēng Tāng* (固卫御风汤) with *shú fù zǐ* （Radix Aconiti Lateralis Praeparata）(processed)

【Ingredients】

黄芪	huáng qí	9g	Radix Astragali
防风	fáng fēng	9g	Radix Saposhnikoviae

炒白术	chǎo bái zhú	9g	Rhizoma Atractylodis Macrocephalae (stir-fried)
桂枝	guì zhī	9g	Ramulus Cinnamomi
赤芍	chì sháo	9g	Radix Paeoniae Rubra
白芍	bái sháo	9g	Radix Paeoniae Alba
生姜	shēng jiāng	3pieces	Rhizoma Zingiberis Recens
大枣	dà zǎo	7	Fructus Jujubae
熟附子	shú fù zǐ	3g	Radix Aconiti Lateralis Praeparata (processed)

(3) Spleen and Stomach pattern

This is the same as Intestine and Stomach urticaria caused by deficient Spleen and Stomach with external wind-cold attack. It manifests as skin rashes on the body, poor appetite, abdominal pain and distention, nausea and vomiting, unformed stool, a white or greasy tongue coat, and a wiry and moderate pulse.

【Treatment Principle】 Fortify the Spleen and regulate qi, course wind and scatter coldness.

【Prescription】

苍术	cāng zhú	9g	Rhizoma Atractylodis
陈皮	chén pí	6g	Pericarpium Citri Reticulatae
茯苓	fú líng	9g	Poria
泽泻	zé xiè	9g	Rhizoma Alismatis
荆芥	jīng jiè	9g	Herba Schizonepetae
羌活	qiāng huó	9g	Rhizoma et Radix Notopterygii
木香	mù xiāng	3g	Radix Aristolochiae
乌药	wū yào	9g	Radix Linderae
生姜	shēng jiāng	3pieces	Rhizoma Zingiberis Recens
大枣	dà zǎo	5	Fructus Jujubae

(4) Blood-heat pattern

This is often seen in artificial urticaria (dermographic disease). In Chinese medicine, it is called *fēng yǐn zhěn* (风隐疹) - wind dormant papules. It is caused by fire in Heart meridian, and blood heat engendering wind.

At the onset, there are few skin lesions. At night, there can be burning sensations and stabbing itching, followed by red and purple lines or patches after scratching. These marks increase with scratching. This is accompanied by vexation and irritability. The tongue body is red, and there is a thin yellow coat. The pulse is wiry, slippery and rapid.

【Treatment Principle】 Cool blood and clear heat, disperse wind and stop itching.

【Prescription】

生地	shēng dì	30g	Radix Rehmanniae Recens
当归	dāng guī	9g	Radix Angelicae Sinensis
荆芥	jīng jiè	9g	Herba Schizonepetae
蝉衣	chán yī	6g	Periostracum Cicadae
苦参	kǔ shēn	9g	Radix Sophorae Flavescentis
白蒺藜	bái jí lí	9g	Fructus Tribuli
知母	zhī mǔ	9g	Rhizoma Anemarrhenae
生石膏	shēng shí gāo	30g	Gypsum Fibrosum
生甘草	shēng gān cǎo	6g	Radix et Rhizoma Glycyrrhizae

(5) Blood stagnation pattern

This pattern is caused by stasis blocking the channels and passageways, the *ying* and *wei qi* not diffusing, and wind heat or wind cold mutually contending. This manifests as dark red skin rashes, a dim complexion, purple lips, and skin rashes on the waistline or around the area where a watch-band is worn. The tongue body is purple and dim, and the pulse is thready and choppy.

【Treatment Principle】 Invigorate the blood and dispel wind.

【Prescription】

当归尾	dāng guī wěi	9g	Radix Angelicae Sinensis
赤芍	chì sháo	9g	Radix Paeoniae Rubra
桃仁	táo rén	9g	Semen Juglandis
红花	hóng huā	9g	Flos Carthami

荆芥	jīng jiè	9g	Herba Schizonepetae
蝉衣	chán yī	6g	Periostracum Cicadae
白蒺藜	bái jí lí	9g	Fructus Tribuli
甘草	gān cǎo	6g	Radix et Rhizoma Glycyrrhizae

(Guang An Men Hospital of Chinese Medicine Researching Institute: Editor-in-chief. *Clinical Experience' Recordings of Zhu Renkang- the Category of Dermal Surgery* 朱仁康临床经验集·皮肤外科. The People's Medical Publishing House, 1979：117)

2. Zhao Bing-nan's four pattern differentiations in the treatment of urticaria — cold, heat, and deficiency patterns with the emphasis on wind evil.

According to his many years of clinical experience, Zhao Bing-nan divided urticaria into 4 treatment patterns, with an emphasis on dispelling wind evil.

(1) Wind-heat pattern (Mainly seen in acute urticaria)

Flat skin rashes occur on exposed areas or over the whole body. They are only slightly higher than the skin, and are red or pink, with severe pruritus. This is accompanied by headache, fever, vexation, thirst, dry stool, and red urine. The tongue body is red, with a thin white or greasy white coat, and a slippery and rapid pulse.

【Treatment Principle】 Treat with pungent and cool herbs to release the exterior, course wind and stop itching.

【Prescription】#1:

荆芥穗	jīng jiè suì	6g	Spica Schizonepetae
防风	fáng fēng	6g	Radix Saposhnikoviae
金银花	jīn yín huā	12g	Flos Lonicerae Japonicae
牛蒡子	niú bàng zǐ	9g	Fructus Arctii
丹皮	dān pí	6g	Cortex Moutan
浮萍	fú píng	6g	Herba Spirodelae

生地	shēng dì	9g	Radix Rehmanniae Recens
薄荷	bò hé	4.5g	Herba Menthae
黄芩	huáng qín	9g	Radix Scutellariae
蝉衣	chán yī	3g	Periostracum Cicadae
生甘草	shēng gān cǎo	6g	Radix et Rhizoma Glycyrrhizae

【Prescription】 #2:

桑叶	sāng yè	9g	Folium Mori
菊花	jú huā	9g	Flos Chrysanthemi
杏仁泥	xìng rén ní	4.5g	Semen Armeniacae Amarum (grinded)
连翘	lián qiào	9g	Fructus Forsythiae
金银花	jīn yín huā	12g	Flos Lonicerae Japonicae
薄荷	bò hé	4.5g	Herba Menthae
甘草	gān cǎo	9g	Radix et Rhizoma Glycyrrhizae
丹皮	dān pí	9g	Cortex Moutan
防风	fáng fēng	9g	Radix Saposhnikoviae

(2) Wind-cold pattern (Mainly seen in chronic urticaria)

Flat skin rashes are spread over the whole body. They are pink-white or pink, and are accompanied by pruritus and aggravated by wind and cold. They can also be accompanied by fever, aversion to cold, diaphoresis, general aching, no thirst, a white tongue coat, and floating and tight pulse. This should be treated with pungently flavored and warm herbs, so as to outthrust the exterior, course wind and stop itching.

【Treatment Principle】 Treat with pungently flavored and warm herbs to outthrust the exterior, course wind and stop itching.

【Prescription】

麻黄	má huáng	3g	Herba Ephedrae
杏仁	xìng rén	4.5g	Semen Armeniacae Amarum
干姜	gān jiāng	3g	Rhizoma Zingiberis
防风	fáng fēng	6g	Radix Saposhnikoviae
浮萍	fú píng	4.5g	Herba Spirodelae

白鲜皮	bái xiān pí	15g	Cortex Dictamni
芥穗	jīng jiè suì	6g	Spica Schizonepetae
蝉衣	chán yī	4.5g	Periostracum Cicadae
陈皮	chén pí	9g	Pericarpium Citri Reticulatae
丹皮	dān pí	9g	Cortex Moutan
生甘草	shēng gān cǎo	6g	Radix et Rhizoma Glycyrrhizae

(3) Heat stagnation with wind attack (Mainly seen in acute urticaria)

There can be lingering wheals and nettle rash with repeated reoccurrences. They are white or red. Severe pruritus causes insomnia. This is accompanied by glomus and fullness in the middle and stomach duct, poor appetite, chest oppression, rotten belching and up-surging of gastric acids, gastric discomfort with acid regurgitation, nausea, abdominal pain, constipation, red urine, a white thick or greasy tongue coat, and a deep and choppy pulse.

【Treatment Principle】 Simultaneously address both exterior and interior syndromes.

【Prescription】

防风	fáng fēng	9g	Radix Saposhnikoviae
金银花	jīn yín huā	15g	Flos Lonicerae Japonicae
地肤子	dì fū zǐ	18g	Fructus Kochiae
芥穗	jiè suì	9g	Spica Schizonepetae
大黄	dà huáng	4.5g	Radix et Rhizoma Rhei
厚朴	hòu pò	9g	Cortex Magnoliae Officinalis
云苓	yún líng	9g	Poria
赤芍	chì sháo	9g	Radix Paeoniae Rubra
甘草	gān cǎo	9g	Radix et Rhizoma Glycyrrhizae

(4) Blood deficiency with wind attack (Mainly seen in chronic urticaria)

There are repeated reoccurrences of skin rashes. These rashes are aggravated in the afternoon and at night, but relieved in the morning and late midnight (early morning hours). It can be accompanied by dizziness, heaviness in head, tiredness of the body, insomnia with many dreams, a pale or red moist tongue body without coat, and a deep, thready and moderate pulse.

【Treatment Principle】 Tonify qi, nourish blood, and course and scatter wind evil.

【Prescription】

生地	shēng dì	30g	Radix Rehmanniae Recens
当归	dāng guī	15g	Radix Angelicae Sinensis
赤芍	chì sháo	18g	Radix Paeoniae Rubra
白芍	bái sháo	18g	Radix Paeoniae Alba
首乌	shǒu wū	15g	Radix Polygoni Multiflori
生芪	shēng qí	15g	Radix Astragali
防风	fáng fēng	9g	Radix Saposhnikoviae
芥穗	jiè suì	9g	Spica Schizonepetae
刺蒺藜	cì jí lí	15g	Fructus Tribuli
麻黄	má huáng	9g	Herba Ephedrae

Of the above four patterns, the wind-heat pattern is more acute than the wind-cold pattern. The treatment principle should be mainly to expel wind evil. Therefore choose herbs that are pungent in flavor and have the function of diffusing and expelling. For cases where the external evil doesn't go deeply and the right *qi* is not deficient, the treatment effect is satisfying. However, for wind-cold or deficiency pattern the treatment effect is comparably unsatisfying. In chronic cases, after being cured and having no new skin rashes, it is advisable to continue taking medicine for a long time or taking a patent medicine to prevent reoccurrence. In the period of treatment and after being cured, dietary restrictions should be followed, including avoiding fish, shrimp, spicy foods and alcohol.

(Shan Shu-jian. Editor-in-chief. *Clinical Recordings of Famous Doctors in*

Ancient and Modern China-Category of Surgery 古今名医临证金鉴. 外科卷.
Chinese Medicine Press, 1999.171)

3. Zhou Ming-qi believes that internal and external wind will damage the right qi, therefore the treatment of wind should be included in both internal and external therapies.

Drawing from his long-term clinical experience, Zhou believes that stubborn urticaria is mainly a transformation of acute urticaria. It is characterized by repeated reoccurrences of skin rashes with severe pruritus. Most cases are accompanied by dizziness, headache, insomnia, numerous dreams, sore lumbar area, and fatigue. For many patients the onset is at a specific time, such as in the spring, autumn, or in the morning or at night. It can also be linked to the menstrual cycle. According to Chinese medical theory, it is caused mainly by deficient yin and blood, internal heat due to yin deficiency, and wind due to blood deficiency. In addition, repeated reoccurrences can result in qi and blood consumption leading to wind attack. Because of the long course of disease, the wind evil can go deep into the *ying* level, blood aspects, and organ systems. This disease can also be caused by disharmony of the *Chong* and *Ren* vessels, and depression of the Liver. In those cases, the treatment should be to dispel evils, while at the same time tonifying the right *qi*. It is necessary to differentiate yin and yang, and excess and deficiency, in order to cautiously to regulate yin and yang, *ying* and *wei*. At the same time it is necessary to consolidate the *wei* and to protect the body from wind.

For blood deficiency, the treatment should be to tonify qi and nourish blood.

Use following medicinals:

生芪	shēng qí	Radix Astragali
党参	dǎng shēn	Radix Codonopsis
当归	dāng guī	Radix Angelicae Sinensis

生地	shēng dì	Radix Rehmanniae Recens
白芍	bái sháo	Radix Paeoniae Alba
川芎	chuān xiōng	Rhizoma Chuanxiong
首乌	shǒu wū	Radix Polygoni Multiflori

For blood stagnation, the treatment should be to move the blood and resolve blood stasis.

Use following medicinals:

桃仁	táo rén	Semen Persicae
红花	hóng huā	Flos Carthami
丹参	dān shēn	Radix et Rhizoma Salviae Miltiorrhizae
鸡血藤	jī xuè téng	Caulis Spatholobi

For wind accompanying these patterns, the treatment should be to course the exterior and dispelling wind.

Use following medicinals:

荆芥	jīng jiè	Herba Schizonepetae
防风	fáng fēng	Radix Saposhnikoviae
刺蒺藜	cì jí lí	Fructus Tribuli

For lingering wind evil treated with no effect by a wind-coursing method, treatment should be to track wind.

Use following medicinals:

蝉蜕	chán tuì	Periostracum Cicadae
僵蚕	jiāng cán	Bombyx Batryticatus
蜈蚣	wú gōng	Scolopendra
乌蛇	wū shé	Zaocys

For disharmony of the *Chong* and *Ren* vessels caused by menstruation, the treatment should be to regulate the *Chong* and *Ren* vessels, and harmonize the qi and blood.

Use following medicinals:

寸云	cùn yún	Herba Cistanches
仙灵脾	xiān líng pí	Epimedium brevicornum Maxim
巴戟	bā jǐ	Radix Morindae Officinalis
柴胡	chái hú	Radix Bupleuri
当归	dāng guī	Radix Angelicae Sinensis
川芎	chuān xiōng	Rhizoma Chuanxiong
赤芍	chì sháo	Radix Paeoniae Rubra
生地	shēng dì	Radix Rehmanniae Recens
丹参	dān shēn	Radix et Rhizoma Salviae Miltiorrhizae

For a lingering course of disease without cure that is aggravated by mental stress and depression, one should treat by calming the spirit.

Use following medicinals:

枣仁	zǎo rén	Semen Ziziphi Spinosae
夜交藤	yè jiāo téng	Caulis Polygoni Multiflori
合欢花	hé huān huā	Flos Albiziae

For heat retention in the Stomach and Intestines with steaming of the skin and dry stools, the treatment should be to moisten and relax the bowels, and purge heat by draining the turbid.

Use following herbs:

瓜蒌仁	guā lóu zǐ rén	Semen Trichosanthis
麻仁	má rén	Fructus Cannabis
首乌	shǒu wū	Radix Polygoni Multiflori

In addition, *kǔ shēn* (Radix Sophorae Flavescentis), *bái xiān pí* (Cortex Dictamni), and *dì fū zǐ* (Fructus Kochiae) can clear heat and drain dampness, expel wind, resolve toxin and stop itching are often used to treat this disease.

(Shi Yu-guang et al, Editors-in-Chief: *Essentials Of Modern Chinese Medicine Doctors' Clinics: Dermatology* 当代名医临证精华·皮肤病专辑. Ancient Books of Chinese Medicine Publishing Office, 1992.104.)

4. Liu Xue-qin treats urticaria mainly by dispersing food (accumulation), abducting stagnation, coursing wind and scattering cold.

Liu Xue-qin believes that the onset of urticaria is closely related to wind, dampness and food retention. In clinic the empirical prescription *Xiāo Zhěn Yī Hào* (消疹一号) is often used to treat the pattern of dampness retained in the Middle Jiao with wind-cold attacking the exterior.

【Prescription】

净蝉蜕	jìng chán tuì	12g	Periostracum Cicadae
独活	dú huó	7g	Radix Angelicae Pubescentis
防风	fáng fēng	9g	Radix Saposhnikoviae
荆芥	jīng jiè	9g	Herba Schizonepetae
地肤子	dì fū zǐ	30g	Fructus Kochiae
焦槟榔	jiāo bīng láng	7g	Semen Arecae Praepareta
草红花	cǎo hóng huā	12g	Flos Carthami
白鲜皮	bái xiān pí	12g	Cortex Dictamni
皂角刺	zào jiǎo cì	7g	Spina Gleditsiae

【Modifications】

For severe disease conditions with lingering pruritus, add *quán xiē* (Scorpio) 8g and *chǎo cì wèi pí* (Erinaceus stir-fried) 12g.

For stomachache with difficult eating, add *chǎo zhǐ qiào* (dry-fried Fructus Aurantii) 12g and *chuān hòu pò* (Cortex Magnoliae Officinalis) 9g.

For gastric and abdominal distention and pain, vexation, and restlessness, add *chǎo zhǐ qiào* (dry-fried Fructus Aurantii) 9g and *shēng dà huáng* (Radix et Rhizoma Rhei) 9g （decocted at the end）.

For bright-red skin rashes with pruritus and a burning sensation on the rashes, add *jīng chì sháo* (Radix Paeoniae Rubra) 12g and *fěn dān pí* (Cortex Moutan) 12g.

For a lingering course of disease without cure, and blood deficiency due to the long-term disease, add *quán dāng guī* (Radix Angelicae Sinensis) 12g and *zhēng shú dì* (Radix Rehmanniae Praeparata) 12g.

For qi deficiency, add *huáng qí* (Radix Astragali) 12g and *míng dǎng shēn* (Radix Changii) 9g.

This method has been used in the clinic for over 20 years, and has been used to treat over one hundred patients, with satisfying results.

【Case Study】 Yang, a 17 year old male, suffered from urticaria for about 10 years. Every year he had several outbreaks. In the early spring there were flare ups. He was treated with Chinese medicine and biomedicine but was not cured. In the evening before this visit, he felt unwell in his stomach and gastric area, and had whole-body dry pruritus. This was followed by thin flat spots of differing sizes gathering together. These spots appeared red around the margins and white in the center. He also had unbearable pruritus, vexation and agitation, stomach fullness and poor appetite, and nausea with a desire to vomit. On his lips and eyelids he had severe edema that resembled pigs' lips.

Use modified *Xiāo Zhěn Yī Hào* (消疹一号).

【Ingredients】

地肤子	dì fū zǐ	30g	Fructus Kochiae
净蝉蜕	jìng chán tuì	12g	Periostracum Cicadae
皂角刺	zào jiǎo cì	7g	Spina Gleditsiae
荆芥	jīng jiè	9g	Herba Schizonepetae
防风	fáng fēng	9g	Radix Saposhnikoviae
槟榔	bīng láng	7g	Semen Arecae
独活	dú huó	7g	Radix Angelicae Pubescentis
全蝎	quán xiē	9g	Scorpio
炒枳壳	chǎo zhǐ qiào	9g	Fructus Aurantii (stir-fried)
川厚扑	chuān hòu pò	9g	Cortex Magnoliae Officinalis
白鲜皮	bái xiān pí	14g	Cortex Dictamni
草红花	cǎo hóng huā	12g	Flos Carthami

After one dose, the lips and eyelids returned to normal. At this moment, it was very important to continue the treatment, so the previous prescription was continued for other 3 doses. It was then modified by adding *shēng huáng qí* (raw Radix Astragali) 12g and *chǎo zhǐ qiào* (dry-fried Fructus Aurantii) 9g. One dose was taken every two days. After a total of 14 doses, the patient was cured and had no reoccurrences during 18 years worth of follow-ups.

According to modern pharmacologic analyses *jīng jiè* (Herba Schizonepetae), *fáng fēng* (Radix Saposhnikoviae), *dì fū zǐ* (Fructus Kochiae), *chán tuì* (Periostracum Cicadae) and *bái xiān pí* (Cortex Dictamni) have good desensitization effects. There are several points that should be noted. A) Indigestion is a main cause for this disease, so along with expelling wind and desensitizing the body, one should also promote digestion and resolve food stagnation. B) Avoid stimulating food like chicken, duck, fish, shrimp, milk, eggs, and spicy foods - even after being cured. C) Avoid wind-cold. D) Take another 3-20 doses after being cured in order to prevent reoccurrences.

(Song Zu-jing, Editor-in-chief. *Clinical Recordings of Modern Famous Doctors* 当代名医证治汇粹. Shi jiazhuang: Hebei Science and Technology Publishing house, 1990.473)

5. Xi Feng-lin believes that the pattern differentiation and corresponding treatment of urticaria should include deficiency and excess patterns.

The famous doctor Xi Feng-lin treated urticaria based on the Liver and obtained some treatment effects. The pattern differentiated is as follows:

(1) Excess patterns:

1) Liver qi stagnation:

Repeated onset of skin rashes aggravated by depression, irritability, and fatigue, often accompanied with oppressive sighing, hypochondriac pain and soreness, a thin tongue coat and a wiry pulse. This should be treated by coursing the Liver and regulating qi.

The commonly used herbs:

柴胡	chái hú	Radix Bupleuri
赤芍	chì sháo	Radix Paeoniae Rubra
枳壳	zhǐ qiào	Fructus Aurantii
香附	xiāng fù	Rhizoma Cyperi
川芎	chuān xiōng	Rhizoma Chuanxiong
生甘草	shēng gān cǎo	raw Radix et Rhizoma Glycyrrhizae
菊花	jú huā	Flos Chrysanthemi
薄荷	bò hé	Herba Menthae

2) Liver qi stagnation transforming into heat:

There are red wheals with pruritus, dizziness, red eyes, hypochondriac pain, vomiting, bitter taste in the mouth, red tongue margins, a yellow tongue coat, and a wiry and rapid pulse. This should be treated by clearing the Liver and purging fire.

The commonly used herbs:

龙胆草	lóng dǎn cǎo	Radix et Rhizoma Gentianae
黑山栀	hēi shān zhī	Fructus Gardeniae
淡子芩	dàn zǐ qín	Radix Scutellariae
生地黄	shēng dì huáng	raw Radix Rehmanniae Recens
柴胡	chái hú	Radix Bupleuri
菊花	jú huā	Flos Chrysanthemi
白蒺藜	bái jí lí	Fructus Tribuli
金银花	jīn yín huā	Flos Lonicerae Japonicae
生甘草	shēng gān cǎo	raw Radix et Rhizoma Glycyrrhizae

3) Liver fire with Intestine dryness:

There are bright red wheals with pruritus, headache, red eyes, irritability, bitter taste in the mouth, dry pharynx, hypochondriac and abdominal pain, constipation, burning pain around the anus, a red tongue, a yellow tongue coat, and a wiry, slippery and rapid pulse. This should be treated by clearing the Liver, opening the *fu* (organs), and resolving both the exterior and interior.

The commonly used herbs:

防风	fáng fēng	Radix Saposhnikoviae
薄荷	bò hé	Herba Menthae
连翘	lián qiào	Fructus Forsythiae
金银花	jīn yín huā	Flos Lonicerae Japonicae
当归	dāng guī	Radix Angelicae Sinensis
赤芍	chì sháo	Radix Paeoniae Rubra
淡子芩	dàn zǐ qín	Radix Scutellariae
桔梗	jié gěng	Radix Platycodonis
生甘草	shēng gān cǎo	Radix et Rhizoma Glycyrrhizae
大黄	dà huáng	Radix et Rhizoma Rhei
芒硝	máng xiāo	Natrii Sulfas

For constipation, add *Gēng Yī Piàn* (更衣片), 2 pills 3 times a day.

(2) Deficiency patterns:

1) Yin and blood deficiency:

There are pale red skin rashes with pruritus, dizziness, depression, dull pain in the hypochondriac region, a red tongue, a dry mouth, and a thin, wiry or rapid pulse. It should be treated by nourishing blood and softening the Liver.

The commonly used herbs：

生地黄	shēng dì huáng	Radix Rehmanniae Recens
当归	dāng guī	Radix Angelicae Sinensis
枸杞子	gǒu qǐ zǐ	Fructus Lycii
川楝子	chuān liàn zǐ	Fructus Toosendan
桑叶	sāng yè	Folium Mori
菊花	jú huā	Flos Chrysanthemi
赤芍	chì sháo	Radix Paeoniae Rubra
白蒺藜	bái jí lí	Fructus Tribuli
醋炒青皮	cù chǎo qīng pí	vinegar-fried Pericarpium Citri Reticulatae Viride

2) Disharmony of *Chong* and *Ren* vessels:

The skin rash often occurs before menstruation, or is aggravated during menstruation, and then subsides after menstruation. It is often accompanied by distending pain in the chest and abdomen, irritability, irregular or scanty menstruation, a thin tongue coat, a wiry pulse, and a dim complexion. It should be treated by regulating the *Chong* and *Ren* vessels.

The commonly used herbs：

桃仁	táo rén	Semen Persicae
红花	hóng huā	Flos Carthami
川芎	chuān xiōng	Rhizoma Chuanxiong
当归	dāng guī	Radix Angelicae Sinensis
生地黄	shēng dì huáng	Radix Rehmanniae Recens
白芍	bái sháo	Radix Paeoniae Alba
制香附	zhì xiāng fù	Rhizoma Cyperi processed
芫蔚子	chōng wèi zǐ	Fructus Leonuri

For excessive menstruation, remove *táo rén* (Semen Persicae), *hóng huā* (Flos Carthami) and *chōng wèi zǐ* (Fructus Leonuri), and add *pào hēi jiāng* (Rhizoma Zingiberis), *zhì gān cǎo* (Radix et Rhizoma Glycyrrhizae Praeparata cum Melle) and *wū yào* (Radix Linderae).

For a distending sensation in the chest with subcutaneous nodules and pain with touch, add *chái hú* (Radix Bupleuri) and *Shī Xiào Sǎn* (失笑散).

For abdominal pain, add *jīn líng zǐ* (Fructus Toosendan) and *yán hú suǒ* (Rhizoma Corydalis).

3) Deficiency of qi and blood:

This is seen mainly in patients with weak constitutions. There are pale or white wheals that turn red after being scratched. There are repeated reoccurrences that can linger for several years without cure, and are aggravated by fatigue. The complexion is pale, and there is poor appetite, fatigue, sleepiness, a thin and moist tongue coat, and a soggy and thin pulse. This should be treated by regulating qi and blood.

The commonly used herbs are:

生黄芪	shēng huáng qí	raw Radix Astragali
白术	bái zhú	Rhizoma Atractylodis Macrocephalae
党参	dǎng shēn	Radix Codonopsis
当归	dāng guī	Radix Angelicae Sinensis
炙甘草	zhì gān cǎo	Radix et Rhizoma Glycyrrhizae Praeparata cum Melle
广木香	guǎng mù xiāng	Radix Aristolochiae
桂圆肉	guì yuán ròu	Arillus Longan
白芍	bái sháo	Radix Paeoniae Alba
生地黄	shēng dì huáng	Radix Rehmanniae Recens
粉丹皮	fěn dān pí	powdered Cortex Moutan

4) Yin deficiency of the Liver and Kidney:

There are irregular flare-ups and remissions of diffused skin rashes, flushed cheekbones, dizziness, sore and weak sensations in the lumbar area and knees, vexation, night sweats, a red tongue without a coat, and a thin and rapid pulse. This should be treated by tonifying the Kidney *yin* so as to moisten the Liver.

The commonly used herbs：

生地黄	shēng dì huáng	Radix Rehmanniae Recens
丹皮	dān pí	Cortex Moutan
山萸肉	shān yú ròu	Fructus Corni
怀山药	huái shān yào	Rhizoma Dioscorea
制首乌	zhì shǒu wū	prepared Radix Polygoni Multiflori
炙龟甲	zhì guī jiǎ	prepared Carapax et Plastrum Testudinis
黄柏	huáng bǎi	Cortex Phellodendri Chinensis
赤芍	chì sháo	Radix Paeoniae Rubra
沙苑子	shā yuàn zǐ	Semen Astragali Complanati
生牡蛎	shēng mǔ lì	Concha Ostreae

The above mentioned patterns mainly pertain to chronic urticaria. The following herbs can be added according to pattern differentiation.

For external wind attacking, add:

荆芥	jīng jiè	Herba Schizonepetae
防风	fáng fēng	Radix Saposhnikoviae
薄荷	bò hé	Herba Menthae
桔梗	jié gěng	Radix Platycodonis
羌活	qiāng huó	Rhizoma et Radix Notopterygii
独活	dú huó	Radix Angelicae Pubescentis
蝉衣	chán yī	Periostracum Cicadae
牛蒡子	niú bàng zǐ	Fructus Arctii

For allergies to foods and medicines, the air and some and flavors, add:

紫苏	zǐ sū	Folium Perillae
僵蚕	jiāng cán	Bombyx Batryticatus
蝉蜕	chán tuì	Periostracum Cicadae
地龙	dì lóng	Pheretima
全蝎	quán xiē	Scorpio
乌蛸蛇	wū shāo shé	Zaocys
苦参	kǔ shēn	Radix Sophorae Flavescentis

For parasite-induced malnutrition, add:

使君子	shǐ jūn zǐ	Fructus Quisqualis
雷丸	léi wán	Omphalia
榧子	fěi zǐ	Semen Torreyae
南瓜子	nǎn guā zǐ	Semen Moschatae
槟榔	bīng láng	Semen Arecae

For lingering pruritus, add:

白鲜皮	bái xiān pí	Cortex Dictamni
地肤子	dì fū zǐ	Fructus Kochiae
乌梅	wū méi	Fructus Mume

| 土荆皮 | tǔ jīng pí | Cortex Pseudolaricis |
| 蛇床子 | shé chuáng zǐ | Fructus Cnidii |

(Song Zu-jing: Editor-in-chief. *Clinical Recordings of Modern Famous Doctors* 当代名医证治汇粹 .Shijiazhuang: Hebei Science and Technology Publishing house, 1990.469)

6. Gu Pi-rong treats stubborn urticaria by the four methods of dispelling, dispersing, extinguishing, and controlling.

Gu believes that stubborn urticaria is caused mainly by an external attack by pathogenic wind or internal wind due to a long-term illness. When it is in the early stage, wind-toxin accumulates in the interstitial spaces and blood vessels, and thus should be treated by dispelling external wind. For a lingering wind-toxin causing the Liver to consume *ying* and blood leading to deficiency of Liver *yin* and internal wind, the treatment should be to calm and extinguish internal wind. The treatments are different according to different pathogeneses. These self-composed four-step therapies include dispelling, dispersing, extinguishing and controlling wind. Using these methods, Gu obtained satisfying results. These methods are discussed in brief as follows:

(1) Early stage wind-dampness accumulating in the interstitial spaces should be treated by dispelling wind, invigorating blood, and dispersing both the interior and exterior levels.

Early stage wind-dampness accumulation in the interstitial spaces externally can have two causative factors: a) loose interstitial spaces due to sweating. b) food retention in the Intestines and Stomach. The combination of an external evil with internal stagnation leads to disharmony of *ying* and *wei,* manifesting as skin rashes with severe pruritus and an indescribable uncomfortable sensation in the stomach region and abdomen, a thin-greasy tongue coat, and a soggy and slippery pulse. A famous doctor, You Zai-jing, once said that "insidious rashes with pruritus are caused by blood disturbed by wind". Therefore the treatment should be to dispel wind, invigorate blood, and disperse the interior and exterior levels. When wind is dispelled, the blood will not be disturbed; when the interior is harmonious, the external evil can not attack. The insidious rashes can be cured by treating from both the exterior and the interior.

【Prescription】

浮萍	fú píng	6g	Herba Spirodelae
炒牛蒡	chǎo niú bàng	9g	Fructus Arctii (stir-fried)
蝉衣	chán yī	6g	Periostracum Cicadae
晚蚕沙	wǎn cán shā	15g	Faeces Bombycis
槟榔	bīng láng	12g	Semen Arecae
白鲜皮	bái xiān pí	15g	Cortex Dictamni
炒枳壳	chǎo zhǐ qiào	12g	Fructus Aurantii (stir-fried)
土茯苓	tǔ fú líng	30g	Rhizoma Smilacis Glabrae
炒赤芍	chǎo chì sháo	12g	Radix Paeoniae Rubra
丹皮	dān pí	9g	Cortex Moutan
生甘草	shēng gān cǎo	6g	Radix et Rhizoma Glycyrrhizae (raw)
防风通圣丸	*Fáng Fēng Tōng Shèng Wán*	12g	

(2) Lingering wind evil attacking the collaterals and should be treated by dispersing wind, harmonizing blood, and coursing and nourishing.

The disease lingers for several months, and even after taking herbs which have the function of dispelling wind, resolving stagnation, harmonizing *ying* and cooling blood, there is still the same amount of pruritus with dry skin. It is aggravated at night, and is accompanied by dizziness, dry stool, a red tongue with a thin coat, and a wiry and thin pulse. This is external wind accumulating in the interstitial spaces and gradually moving into the blood vessels. Blood belongs to yin, as does the night, so the disease is aggravated at night. The thin and greasy tongue coat shows that there is a remaining external evil. The dry skin and dizziness indicates blood and *ying* deficiency. The treatment should be to disperse wind and harmonize blood. "Treatment of wind should be based on the treatment of blood, and the wind can be calmed by moving the blood."

【Prescription】

豨草	xiān cǎo	15g	Herba Siegesbeckiae
炒牛蒡	chǎo niú bàng	9g	Fructus Arctii (stir-fried)
蝉衣	chán yī	6g	Periostracum Cicadae
晚蚕沙	wǎn cán shā	15g	Faeces Bombycis
白蒺藜	bái jí lí	12g	Fructus Tribuli
当归	dāng guī	12g	Radix Angelicae Sinensis
生地黄	shēng dì huáng	15g	Radix Rehmanniae Recens
炒赤芍	chǎo chì sháo	12g	Radix Paeoniae Rubra (stri-fried)
丹皮	dān pí	9g	Cortex Moutan
生甘草	shēng gān cǎo	6g	Radix et Rhizoma Glycyrrhizae (raw)
白鲜皮	bái xiān pí	15g	Cortex Dictamni
生首乌	shēng shǒu wū	15g	Radix Polygoni Multiflori
木通	mù tōng	3g	Caulis Akebiae
土茯苓	tǔ fú líng	30g	Rhizoma Smilacis Glabrae

(3) In the case of long-term illness with ying deficiency and wind, the treatment should be to extinguish wind and nourish blood. Attention should be paid to both clearing and nourishing.

These cases of urticaria linger for over a year, accompanied by dry skin, dizziness, headache, and irritability even after being treated (without effect) by eliminating wind, transforming dampness, harmonizing *ying* and invigorating blood. This is because wind *qi* internally moves in the Liver, and wind that comes from the exterior lingers without resolution. Therefore internally the yin and blood are consumed, and formulas to dispel wind that are taken over a long time can also disperse and scorch the Liver and *ying*. In cases of urticaria that last for many years, although the exterior wind is resolved, the Liver *yin* is damaged and deficiency wind is internally engendered. As a result, the tongue is red with little coat and the pulse is deficient and wiry. This is a manifestation of less evil and more deficiency. It seems that herbs that are acrid and scattering not only consume *ying*, but also cause even more skin rashes. The treatment should extinguish wind and nourish blood, with effects seen over a long course of time.

【Prescription】

天麻	tiān má	6g	Rhizoma Gastrodiae
钩藤	gōu téng	12g	Ramulus Uncariae Cum Uncis
桑叶	sāng yè	12g	Folium Mori
白蒺藜	bái jí lí	12g	Fructus Tribuli
当归	dāng guī	12g	Radix Angelicae Sinensis
生地黄	shēng dì huáng	15g	Radix Rehmanniae Recens
炒白芍	chǎo bái sháo	10g	Radix Paeoniae Alba (dry-fried)
制首乌	zhì shǒu wū	12g	Radix Polygoni Multiflori (processed)
胡麻仁	hú má rén	15g	Fructus Cannabis
煅龙骨	duàn lóng gǔ	12g	Os Draconis（calcined）
煅牡蛎	duàn mǔ lì	12g	Concha Ostreae（calcined）
山药	shān yào	20g	Rhizoma Dioscoreae
穞豆衣	lǔ dòu yī	12g	Spermodermis Phaseoli Radiati

(4) For long-term urticaria induced by cold, the treatment should be to resist wind and substantiate the *wei*, nourish *ying* and consolidate the exterior.

This is long-standing urticaria that occurs regularly on freezing cold days on exposed areas of the body, such as the head, face and four limbs. When exposed to cold wind, wheals occur suddenly, accompanied by severe pruritus. They disappear in the warm spring. This can be accompanied by pale complexion, aversion to cold, freezing and numbness of the four limbs, dizziness, a pale tongue body, a thin white coat, and a soggy and thin pulse. This is caused by long-term disease leading to qi and blood deficiency. When *ying* is weak internally, *wei* can not circulate normally. This leads to blood stasis in the collaterals. It is commonly believed that there are wind and cold internal and external evils that cause urticaria. Although this is a minor illness, it is usually difficult to achieve results with treatment. It is suitable to use a large formula to regulate and guard the *wei* and yang so as to control deficient wind. Tonify and nourish the *ying* and yin so as to open the blood vessels. When the *ying* and blood are regulated through treatment, the qi and blood have harmonious flow and therefore it is difficult for wind and cold to attack, then how can urticaria occur?

【Prescription】

生芪	shēng qí	20g	Radix Astragali
焦白术	jiāo bái zhú	15g	Rhizoma Atractylodis Macrocephalae (charred)
防风	fáng fēng	6g	Radix Saposhnikoviae
桂枝	guì zhī	9g	Ramulus Cinnamomi
炒赤芍	chǎo chì sháo	9g	Radix Paeoniae Rubra （dry-fried）
炒白芍	chǎo bái sháo	9g	Radix Paeoniae Alba （dry-fried）
当归	dāng guī	15g	Radix Angelicae Sinensis
细辛	xì xīn	3g	Radix et Rhizoma Asari
木通	mù tōng	6g	Caulis Akebiae
红花	hóng huā	6g	Flos Carthami
川芎	chuān xiōng	9g	Rhizoma Chuanxiong
炙甘草	zhì gān cǎo	6g	Radix et Rhizoma Glycyrrhizae Praeparata cum Melle
鲜生姜	xiān shēng jiāng	3pieces	Rhizoma Zingiberis Recens
红枣	hóng zǎo	7pieces	Fructus Jujubae
陈绍酒		1cup	wine

(Shi Yu-guang et al, Editors-in-Chief: *Essentials Of Modern Chinese Medicine Doctors' Clinic: Dermatosis* 当代名医临证精华 . 皮肤病专辑 . Ancient Books of Chinese Medicine Publishing Office, 1992. 86.)

7. He Ren treats urticaria by coursing wind and resolving toxin.

He believes that urticaria is caused mainly by sweating in the presence of wind. Then the exterior evil invades the interstices. Wind qi transforms in the flesh and skin and becomes mutually bound with heat. In acute cases, the skin rashes will last 1-2 days or 4-5days. In chronic cases, the skin rashes disappear several days later but reoccur over a lingering course of diseases. In severe cases, the disease course can last for several months or years and transform into a stubborn illness. The treatment should always be to course wind, resolve toxin, clear heat, and purge fire. This pattern can be differentiated from qi and blood aspects and treated with a basic prescription modified according to the pattern. The basic formula is *Má Huáng Lián Qiào Chì Xiǎo Dòu Tāng*, as recorded in *Discussion of Cold Damage*. When it is in the early stage and located in the exterior, *guì zhī* (Ramulus Cinnamomi) and *fú píng* (Herba Spirodelae) can be added. For a lingering course of disease, *hēi zhī ma* (Semen Sesami Nigri) 30g, *hé shǒu wū* (Radix Polygoni Multiflori) 9g, *kǔ shēn* (Radix Sophorae Flavescentis) 6g, *shí chāng pǔ* (Rhizoma Acori Tatarinowii) 6g and *gān cǎo* (Radix et Rhizoma Glycyrrhizae) 5g can be added. *Huáng jiǔ* (yellow rice wine) 30-60g also can be used for those patients who can drink alcohol 1 dosage per day. The efficacy is obvisous.

If the patients has a lingering course, crimson and mirror-like tongue body, its indicated that the evil have entered into blood collaterals, add:

地龙	dì lóng	9g	Pheretima
刺猬皮	cì wèi pí	9g	Corium Erinacei seu Hemiechini
杏仁	xìng rén	6g	Armeniacae Semen Amarum
赤芍	chì sháo	6g	Radix Paeoniae Rubra
皂角刺	zào jiǎo cì	5g	Spina Gleditsiae

or appropriate amount of

银花	yín huā		Flos Lonicerae Japonicae
薄荷	bò hé		Herba Menthae

Ms. Zhao, 40 years old, being attacked by wind evil during showering after swimming, the skin rash was spread all over the body with different sizes accompanied with itching, burning sensation, insomia, yellow urine, dry stool. The treatment should be dispel damp-heat.

The following herbs were used:

麻黄	má huáng	5g	Herba Ephedrae
连翘	lián qiào	9g	Fructus Forsythiae
赤小豆	chì xiǎo dòu	15g	Semen Phaseoli
黑芝麻	hēi zhī ma	30g	Semen Sesami Nigri
何首乌	hé shǒu wū	9g	Radix Polygoni Multiflori
苦参	kǔ shēn	6g	Radix Sophorae Flavescentis
生甘草	shēng gān cǎo	5g	Radix et Rhizoma Glycyrrhizae (raw)
石菖蒲	shí chāng pú	6g	Rhizoma Acori Tatarinowii
黄酒		30g	yellow wine

After 2 doses the skin rashes will disappear.

(He Ren. Editor-in-Chief: *Clinical Recordings of He Ren* 何任临床经验辑要. Beijing: Chinese Medical Science and Technology Publishing House, 1998.63)

PERSPECTIVES OF INTEGRATIVE MEDICINE

Challenges and Solutions

Based on the course of disease, urticaria can be divided into acute and chronic types. Chronic urticaria has an indefinite and complicated etiology and is hard to cure. It manifests with repeated reoccurrences, bring great physical and emotional pain and inconvenience to the patient. Sudden onset can be severe, with symptoms that can lead to asphyxia and shock, endangering the life of the patient. Therefore preventing and reducing the recurrences of urticaria becomes the challenging clinical task.

Challenge #1: How to Prevent the Onset of Urticaria

Because of its complicated etiology and induction from complex internal and external factors, prevention should be based on two aspects: eliminating allergens and controlling infection.

1) Eliminating the allergen

The onset of urticaria is related to coming in contact with an allergen. Things that can cause urticaria include some proteins like shrimp, crab and other seafood, eggs, mushroom, beans, milk, and bamboo shoots. These should be avoided. Medications that can cause urticaria should be prohibited. In cases of urticaria induced by bacteria, fungal spores, animal dander, feathers, industrial dust, volatile chemicals, the allergen should be avoided. For those cases induced by cold, heat, sunlight and other physical stimulations, the patient should pay attention to changing clothing in accordance with the climate and avoid being directly exposed to sunlight. There should also be good home hygiene so as to eliminate dust, mites and cockroaches that can induce urticaria.

2) Controlling the infection

In some cases, the onset of urticaria is closely related to infection. There are four main types of sources of general infection: parasites, viruses, bacteria and fungi. Chinese medicine achieves satisfying results in the treatment of intestinal parasites. Chinese herbs used include *chuān liàn zǐ* (Fructus Toosendan), *shǐ jūn zǐ* (Fructus Quisqualis), *nán guā zǐ* (Semen Moschatae), *kǔ jǐn pí* (Cortex Hibisci), *léi wán* (Omphalia) and *bīng láng* (Semen Arecae) to kill roundworm, filariasis, hookworm and pinworm, and *qīng hāo* (Herba Artemisiae Annuae), *cháng shān* (Radix

Dichroae) and *bái tóu wēng* (Radix Pulsatillae) to kill plasmodium and amoeba parasites.

To control a viral infection, different herbs can be chosen according to pattern differentiation.

For wind-heat attacking the exterior, herbs which have strong antivirus actions can be chosen from herbs that are pungent in flavor and cool in property.

These include:

金银花	jīn yín huā	Flos Lonicerae Japonicae
薄荷	bò hé	Herba Menthae
连翘	lián qiào	Fructus Forsythiae
木贼	mù zéi	Herba Equiseti Hiemalis
蝉蜕	chán tuì	Periostracum Cicadae

For internally exuberant heat-toxin, use herbs which have antivirus actions, choose from herbs that clear heat and resolve toxin.

These include:

板蓝根	bǎn lán gēn	Radix Isatidis
大青叶	dà qīng yè	Folium Isatidis
蒲公英	pú gōng yīng	Herba Taraxaci
紫草	zǐ cǎo	Radix Arnebiae
马齿苋	mǎ chǐ xiàn	Herba Portulacae

For wind-cold attacking the exterior, choose herbs which have antivirus actions from herbs that are pungent in flavor and warm in property.

These include:

麻黄	má huáng	Herba Ephedrae
桂枝	guì zhī	Ramulus Cinnamomi
苏叶	sū yè	Folium Perillae
荆芥	jīng jiè	Herba Schizonepetae

Pharmacological research on bacterial infection control shows the following results.

For controlling gram-positive bacteria, the following herbs have a good treatment effect.

黄芩	huáng qín	Radix Scutellariae
黄柏	huáng bǎi	Cortex Phellodendri Chinensis
紫花地丁	zǐ huā dì dīng	Herba Violae
蒲公英	pú gōng yīng	Herba Taraxaci
鱼腥草	yú xīng cǎo	Herba Houttuyniae
败酱草	bài jiàng cǎo	Herba Patriniae
丹皮	dān pí	Cortex Moutan

For controlling gram-negative bacteria, the following herbs have a good treatment effect.

射干	shè gān	Rhizoma Belamcandae
秦皮	qín pí	Cortex Fraxini
木香	mù xiāng	Radix Aucklandiae
厚扑	hòu pò	Cortex Magnoliae Officinalis
百部	bǎi bù	Radix Stemonae
白芷	bái zhǐ	Radix Angelicae Dahuricae
丁香	dīng xiāng	Flos Caryophylli
乌梅	wū méi	Fructus Mume

For controlling fungal infection, the following herbs have strong actions:

黄精	huáng jīng	Rhizoma Polygonati
绵茵陈	mián yīn chén	Herba Artemisiae Scopariae
土茯苓	tǔ fú líng	Rhizoma Smilacis Glabrae
丁香	dīng xiāng	Flos Caryophylli
黄连	huáng lián	Rhizoma Coptidis
白鲜皮	bái xiān pí	Cortex Dictamni
地肤子	dì fū zǐ	Fructus Kochiae
甘草	gān cǎo	Radix et Rhizoma Glycyrrhizae

In addition to correlating treatments according to pattern differentiation, proper herbs can be chosen to control infection, eliminate the original cause, and reduce the number of flare-ups.

Challenge #2: How to Reduce the Reoccurrence of Urticaria

Chronic urticaria has complicated etiologies and a long course. It is hard to cure, and there are repeated reoccurrences. Reducing the reoccurrence of urticaria is a clinical challenge.

From a biomedicine perspective, it is essential to eliminate the causative factors of urticaria in order to prevent its reoccurrence. However, this is hard to accomplish. Therefore, this is not a satisfactory method of controlling reoccurrences. The Chinese medicine perspective is that "patterns are differentiated according to etiology, and treatments are based on patterns". Chronic urticaria is caused by the flesh and skin becoming malnourished, and can be from a weak constitution or any of the following conditions: damage of qi and blood due to long-term illness, blood deficiency engendering wind, qi deficiency with the *wei* and exterior not consolidated, wind cold evil overwhelming deficiency and invading, unsmooth emotions, Liver depression, weakness and constant illness, lack of sexual moderation leading to Liver and Kidney depletion and damage, dis-regulation of the *Chong* and *Ren,* and the flesh and skin becoming malnourished. In the clinic, the Chinese medical treatment is based on pattern differentiation and can effectively reduce the reoccurrences.

The biomedical pathogenesis of chronic urticaria is divided into two main types: immune and non-immune. Urticaria that is related to immunity is caused by type I and III allergic reactions and is mainly linked to a type I hypersensitivity. All of the allergic reactions are caused by allergens entering the body and stimulating the mast cells to release histamine. Histamine is the main cause of this disease. Therefore antihistamines are routinely used in biomedicine. However, most biomedical antihistamines have side-effects, like drowsiness. Certain drugs have side effects from long-term use that impact the functioning of organs. Therefore long-term use is prohibited. Chinese medicine has fewer side effects than biomedicine. Based on pattern differentiation, one should choose herbs that have been proven by modern pharmacological tests to have antihistamine and anti-inflammatory effects. These include the following herbs:

荆芥	jīng jiè	Herba Schizonepeta
防风	fáng fēng	Radix Saposhnikoviae
白鲜皮	bái xiān pí	Cortex Dictamni
蝉蜕	chán tuì	Periostracum Cicadae
黄芩	huáng qín	Radix Scutellariae
金银花	jīn yín huā	Flos Lonicerae Japonicae
连翘	lián qiào	Fructus Forsythiae
生石膏	shēng shí gāo	Gypsum Fibrosum
生地黄	shēng dì huáng	Radix Rehmanniae Recens
乌梅	wū méi	Fructus Mume
五味子	wǔ wèi zǐ	Fructus Schisandrae Chinensis
龙骨	lóng gǔ	Os Draconis
牡蛎	mǔ lì	Concha Ostreae

Because in most cases of chronic urticaria the immune function is low, internal and external factors can easily attack the body and cause disease flare-ups. Therefore improving the function of the immune system is an important method used to address reoccurrences of chronic urticaria. Chronic urticaria is commonly differentiated as a deficiency pattern; and is often treated by strengthening the Spleen and tonifying qi, regulating and tonifying the Liver and Kidney, and nourishing blood and dispelling wind. According to pharmacological studies, there are many Chinese medicinals that have the function of improving the body's immunity. These include:

Medicinals for tonifying qi and strengthening the Spleen:

党参	dǎng shēn	Radix Codonopsis
茯苓	fú líng	Poria
白术	bái zhú	Rhizoma Atractylodis Macrocephalae
大枣	dà zǎo	Fructus Jujubae

Medicinals for regulating and nourishing the Liver and Kidney:

山茱萸	shān zhū yú	Fructus Corni
女贞子	nǚ zhēn zǐ	Fructus Ligustri Lucidi
旱莲草	hàn lián cǎo	Herba Ecliptae
菟丝子	tù sī zǐ	Semen Cuscutae
仙灵脾	xiān líng pí	Epimedium brevicornum Maxim
紫河车	zǐ hé chē	Placenta Hominis
蛤蚧	gé jiè	Gecko

Medicinals for nourishing blood and dispelling wind:

当归	dāng guī	Radix Angelicae Sinensis
黄精	huáng jīng	Rhizoma Polygonati
大枣	dà zǎo	Fructus Jujubae
白芍	bái sháo	Radix Paeoniae Alba

The prescriptions commonly used to tonify are: *Bā Zhēn Tāng*, *Yù Píng Fēng Sǎn*, *Guī Pí Wán* (归脾丸), *Liù Wèi Dì Huáng Wán* (六味地黄丸), and *Er Zhì Wán* (二至丸).

Insight from Empirical Wisdom

(1) The Treatment of Urticaria Should be Divided into Acute and Chronic Stages.

Through the experience of long-term clinical practice, it has been realized that urticaria should be divided into two types based on the course of the disease – chronic and acute. Acute urticaria disappears after several days or weeks and it is easy to find the etiology. After eliminating the cause, it quickly disappears. Chinese medicine and biomedicine both have satisfying results in the treatment of acute urticaria. This type is mainly differentiated as a heat and excess pattern. The other most commonly encountered internal patterns are wind-heat, wind due to blood-heat, and damp-heat in the Intestines and Stomach. Wind evil is the main external causative factor and should be treated by coursing wind and stopping itching. Herbs that are used are pungent in flavor and cool in property, release the exterior, clear heat and cool blood, and clear heat and relax the bowels. The prescriptions are pungent in flavor and cool in property and have the function of releasing the exterior.

Here, commonly used formulas include: *Yín Qiào Săn* (银翘散), *Qīng Rè Xiāo Fēng Săn* (清热消风散), and *Má Huáng Lián Qiào Chì Xiăo Dòu Tāng.*

Commonly used herbs include:

荆芥	jīng jiè	Herba Schizonepeta
防风	fáng fēng	Radix Saposhnikoviae
浮萍	fú píng	Herba Spirodelae
蝉蜕	chán tuì	Periostracum Cicadae
桑白皮	sāng bái pí	Cortex Mori
桑叶	sāng yè	Folium Mori
牛子	niú zǐ	Fructus Arctii
薄荷	bò hé	Herba Menthae
苦参	kǔ shēn	Radix Sophorae Flavescentis
徐长卿	xú cháng qīng	Radix et Rhizoma Cynanchi Paniculati
刺蒺藜	cì jí lí	Fructus Tribuli
白鲜皮	bái xiān pí	Cortex Dictamni
地肤子	dì fū zǐ	Fructus Kochiae

The commonly used prescriptions used for clearing heat and cooling blood are *Liáng Xuè Xiāo Fēng Săn* (凉血消风散), *Xī Jiăo Dì Huáng Tāng* (犀角地黄汤), and *Huáng Lián Jiě Dú Tāng* (黄连解毒汤).

Commonly used medicinals include:

金银花	jīn yín huā	Flos Lonicerae Japonicae
黄芩	huáng qín	Radix Scutellariae
黄连	huáng lián	Rhizoma Coptidis
黄柏	huáng bǎi	Cortex Phellodendri Chinensis
水牛角	shuǐ niú jiǎo	Cornu Bubali
鱼腥草	yú xīng cǎo	Herba Houttuyniae
龙胆草	lóng dǎn cǎo	Radix et Rhizoma Gentianae
白茅根	bái máo gēn	Rhizoma Imperatae
茜草根	qiàn cǎo gēn	Radix et Rhizoma Rubiae
生石膏	shēng shí gāo	Gypsum Fibrosum
知母	zhī mǔ	Rhizoma Anemarrhenae
牡丹皮	mǔ dān pí	Cortex Moutan

The commonly used prescriptions for clearing heat and relaxing bowels to remove food retention are *Zhǐ Shí Dǎo Zhì Wán* (枳实导滞丸), *Fáng Fēng Tōng Shèng Sǎn* (防风通圣散) and *Jiàn Pí Wán* (健脾丸).

Commonly used herbs include：

大黄	dà huáng	Radix et Rhizoma Rhei
芒硝	máng xiāo	Natrii Sulfas
冬瓜仁	dōng guā rén	Semen Benincasae
山楂	shān zhā	Fructus Crataegi
槟榔	bīng láng	Semen Arecae
神曲	shén qū	Massa Medicata Fermentata
布渣叶	bù zhā yè	Microcos Paniculata Linn
莱菔子	lái fú zǐ	Semen Raphani

Chronic urticaria is a long course of disease with repeated reoccurrences. It is hard to find its complex etiologies. It is treated mainly with a combination of Chinese medicine and biomedicine. It is usually differentiated as a deficiency and stagnation pattern. The 5 most commonly encountered patterns are as follows. 1) Spleen deficiency with cold evil attacking, with the *wei* and exterior not consolidated. 2) Qi and blood deficiency. 3) Internal wind due to Kidney and Liver *yin* deficiency. 4) Qi stasis and blood stagnation. 5) Disharmony between the *Chong* and *Ren* vessels. Because the symptoms manifest externally but the pathogenesis is internal, the treatment should consider the *wei*, qi and blood levels.

Treatments should be differentiated into the following methods. Nourish the spleen, fortify qi, scatter cold, and consolidate the exterior. Increase qi, nourish blood, course wind, and stop itching. Regulate and tonify the Liver and Kidney, nourish blood, and extinguish wind. Invigorate blood, transform stagnation, dispel wind, and stop itching. Tonify and increase the Liver and Kidney, regulate and contain the *Chong* and *Ren*.

The prescriptions for tonifying qi and nourishing blood, dispelling cold and strengthening the superficial resistance are *Bǔ Zhōng Yì Qì Tāng* (补中益气汤), *Yù Píng Fēng Sǎn*, and *Má Huáng Guì Zhī Gè Bàn Tāng* (麻黄桂技各半汤).

Commonly used herbs include:

黄芪	huáng qí	Radix Astragali
党参	dǎng shēn	Radix Codonopsis
茯苓	fú líng	Poria
白术	bái zhú	Rhizoma Atractylodis Macrocephalae
甘草	gān cǎo	Radix et Rhizoma Glycyrrhizae
大枣	dà zǎo	Fructus Jujubae
生姜	shēng jiāng	Rhizoma Zingiberis Recens
麻黄	má huáng	Herba Ephedrae
桂枝	guì zhī	Ramulus Cinnamomi
苏叶	sū yè	Folium Perillae

The prescriptions for tonifying qi and nourishing blood, dispelling wind and relieving itching are *Bā Zhēn Tāng*, *Dāng Guī Yǐn Zi* (当归饮子), and *Sì Wù Xiāo Fēng Sǎn* (四物消风散).

Commonly used herbs include:

当归	dāng guī	Radix Angelicae Sinensis
生地黄	shēng dì huáng	Radix Rehmanniae Recens
熟地黄	shú dì huáng	Radix Rehmanniae Praeparata
天门冬	tiān mén dōng	Radix Asparagi
麦门冬	mài mén dōng	Radix Ophiopogonis
制首乌	zhì shǒu wū	Radix Polygoni Multiflori Praeparata
黄精	huáng jīng	Rhizoma Polygonati
白芍	bái sháo	Radix Paeoniae Alba
胡麻仁	hú má rén	Fructus Cannabis
刺蒺藜	cì jí lí	Fructus Tribuli

The prescriptions for regulating the Liver and Kidney, nourishing blood and extinguishing wind are *Liù Wèi Dì Huáng Tāng* (六味地黄汤), *Yī Guàn Jiān* (一贯煎), and *Er Jiǎ Tāng* (二甲汤).

Commonly used herbs include:

山茱萸	shān zhū yú	Fructus Corni
蕤仁肉	ruí rén ròu	Prinsepia uniflora Batal
淮山	huái shān	Rhizoma Dioscoreae
生地黄	shēng dì huáng	Radix Rehmanniae Recens
石斛	shí hú	Caulis Dendrobii
枸杞子	gǒu qǐ zǐ	Fructus Lycii
鳖甲	biē jiǎ	Carapax Trionycis
龟甲	guī jiǎ	Carapax et Plastrum Testudinis
地龙	dì lóng	Pheretima
乌梅	wū méi	Fructus Mume
五味子	wǔ wèi zǐ	Fructus Schisandrae Chinensis

The prescriptions for moving blood and resolving blood stasis, dispelling wind and relieving itching are *Huó Xuè Qū Fēng Tāng* (活血祛风汤), *Xuè Fǔ Zhú Yū Tāng* (血府逐瘀汤), and *Táo Hóng Sì Wù Tāng* (桃红四物汤).

Commonly used herbs include:

当归	dāng guī	Radix Angelicae Sinensis
川芎	chuān xiōng	Rhizoma Chuanxiong
白芍	bái sháo	Radix Paeoniae Alba
桃仁	táo rén	Semen Juglandis
红花	hóng huā	Flos Carthami
炮姜	pào jiāng	Rhizoma Zingiberis
牛膝	niú xī	Radix Achyranthis Bidentatae
鸡血藤	jī xuè téng	Caulis Spatholobi
柴胡	chái hú	Radix Bupleuri
桔梗	jié gěng	Radix Platycodonis

The prescriptions for regulating the Liver and Kidney, and the *Chong* and *Ren* vessels are *Er Zhì Wán* (二至丸), and *Jiǔ Yuán Jiān* (举元煎).

The commonly used herbs are:

女贞子	nǚ zhēn zǐ	Fructus Ligustri Lucidi
旱莲草	hàn lián cǎo	Herba Ecliptae
菟丝子	tù sī zǐ	Semen Cuscutae
茺蔚子	chōng wèi zǐ	Fructus Leonuri
升麻	shēng má	Rhizoma Cimicifugae
黄芪	huáng qí	Radix Astragali
白术	bái zhú	Rhizoma Atractylodis Macrocephalae
仙灵脾	xiān líng pí	Epimedium brevicornum Maxim
白芍	bái sháo	Radix Paeoniae Alba
红花	hóng huā	Flos Carthami
肉桂	ròu guì	Cortex Cinnamomi

Biomedicine uses one, or a combination, of antihistamines to treat urticaria. The most commonly used treatments are the combination therapy of H1 and H2 receptor antagonists, or antihistamines in combination with coagulants, vitamin C or vitamin K, in combination with calcium, and anti-asthmatic agents (aminophylline). The combined therapy of Chinese medicine with biomedicine is used to treat the acute attacks of chronic urticaria. When the symptoms are relieved, biomedicines can be reduced gradually. Chinese medicines can be continued for 1-2 months until the disease condition is stable. Using a combination of Chinese medicine and biomedicine is conducive to rapidly relieve symptoms, while at the same time significantly reduce the reoccurrence of urticaria outbreaks.

(2) The Complexity and Changeability of Patterns

The patterns of urticaria are complicated. They are often manifested as deficiency accompanied by stasis, wind-heat accompanied by dampness, or qi deficiency accompanied by wind-cold attack. The deficiency pattern can include Liver, Spleen or Kidney deficiencies, or deficiency of both the Liver and Kidney, deficiency of both the Spleen and Kidney, or deficiency of the Liver, Spleen and Kidney. Therefore, to ensure proper treatment, pattern differentiations should be based upon symptoms and constitution.

In addition, the patterns can transform into each other instead of staying static. For example, acute urticaria in the early stage is caused by external wind-cold attack or wind-heat. With improper treatment or lack of treatment, the disease can linger and cause impairment of the right *qi*, leading to an excess pattern transforming into deficiency pattern. On the other hand, chronic urticaria followed be an attack of external wind-cold or wind-heat can manifest as fever, running nose and cough and should be treated according to the following principle: "for emergency cases it is essential to treat the acute symptoms first and when these are relieved, the fundamental cause needs to be dealt with" First use the methods of coursing wind and scattering cold (or heat) in order to treat the symptoms. Then after the exterior symptoms are relieved, treat the causes. Therefore in the clinic, it is essential to inquire into the history of the illness and observe the pathologic changes in order to make an accurate pattern differentiation and corresponding treatment plan.

(3) The Experience of Using Herbs Which Have the Functions of Moving Blood and Freeing Collaterals.

"Wind is the determinant factor in the cause of various diseases." The onset of urticaria is mostly related to wind evil. In cases of acute urticaria, the wind evil will cause pruritus. According to the idea that "the treatment of wind should be based on the treatment of blood; wind can be calmed by the movement of blood", treatment should be to move blood, dispel wind, and stop itching. For chronic urticaria, the principle that "long-term disease causes stasis" should be addressed, and the treatment should be to move blood and dispel wind. Therefore herbs that move blood play an important role in the treatment of urticaria. For stubborn urticaria that lingers over a long time, the use of herbs that move blood (based on pattern differentiation) achieves a satisfying effect. Modern pharmacological research reveals that herbs with the functions of moving blood and resolving stasis can improve immune function, increase microcirculation, and lower capillary permeability so as to improve anti-inflammatory and anti-allergic effects. Herbs which have the functions of moving blood and resolving stasis should be added based on pattern differentiation.

For heat patterns, add:

赤芍	chì sháo	Radix Paeoniae Rubra
丹参	dān shēn	Radix et Rhizoma Salviae Miltiorrhizae
茜草	qiàn cǎo	Radix et Rhizoma Rubae
白花蛇舌草	bái huā shé shé cǎo	Herba Hedyotis
豨莶草	xī xiān cǎo	Herba Siegesbeckiae

For cold patterns, add:

威灵仙	wēi líng xiān	Radix et Rhizoma Clematidis
乌梢蛇	wū shāo shé	Zaocys

For deficiency patterns, add:

当归	dāng guī	Radix Angelicae Sinensis
川芎	chuān xiōng	Rhizoma Chuanxiong
鸡血藤	jī xuè téng	Caulis Spatholobi

For excess patterns, add:

桃仁	táo rén	Semen Juglandis
红花	hóng huā	Flos Carthami
三棱	sān léng	Rhizoma Sparganii
莪术	é zhú	Rhizoma Curcumae
益母草	yì mǔ cǎo	Herba Leonuri

(4) The Experience of Using *Quán Xiē* (Scorpio) to Treat Chronic Urticaria

Chronic urticaria is caused mainly by long-term disease damaging the yin and blood and leading to internal wind or blood deficiency with wind-cold attacking. *Quán xiē* (Scorpio) has the function of dispelling and extinguishing wind, freeing the collaterals and removing stagnation. It is said to "move without containing, and extinguish internal and external wind". In addition, it has the function of leading the other herbs to the surface, superficial and tertiary collaterals. Because of its obvious functions of dispelling and expelling wind, Li Dong-yuan believed that "*it was an essential herb to treat wind*". It was recorded in *Kai Bao Herbs* (开宝本草 , *Kāi Bǎo Běn Cǎo*) that "*quán xiē* (Scorpio) has the function of treating various kinds of insidious rashes that are caused by wind". Therefore *quán xiē* (Scorpio) can be used to treat chronic urticaria with a satisfying effect. The general dosage is 3-6g, taken with water, 3 times a day. It can also be decocted with other herbs. Because of its toxicity, the first dosage should be small and then gradually increased in accordance with disease severity. For urticaria, the maximum dosage is 9g every day. In addition, because *quán xiē* (Scorpio) belongs to the category of insect products, those allergic to animal proteins such as seafood, fish, and beef or other insect herbs (*like dì lóng* [Pheretima], *chán tuì* [Periostracum Cicadae], *fēng fáng* [Nidus Vespae] and *wú gōng* [Scolopendra]) should take it cautiously.

(5) The Clinical Usage of Some Marvelous Herbs that are Used to Treat Urticaria

Through long-term clinical practice and modern pharmacological research it has been concluded that with proper pattern differentiation, some Chinese medicines, used in combination, can promote treatment effects while controlling toxicity. This is seen in the following examples.

1) *Má huáng* (Herba Ephedrae) and *mǔ lì* (Concha Ostreae) to treat wind-cold chronic urticaria:

Má huáng (Herba Ephedrae) is pungent in flavor and warm in property, and has the functions of coursing and scattering wind-cold, diffusing the Lung, coursing wind and stopping itching, dispelling evils and out thrusting rashes. *Mǔ lì* (Concha Ostreae) is salty in flavor and cold and heavy, with a downward nature. Because of this weightiness, it has the functions of calming mind, calming the Liver and subduing the yang, astringing, and relieving acid hyperactivity so as to relieve pain. The combination of these two herbs has the functions of dispelling wind and releasing the exterior, astringing yin and stopping itching. The astringing function of *mǔ lì* (Concha Ostreae) can restrain the hyperactive and dispelling nature of *má huáng* (Herba Ephedrae). According to modern pharmacological research, *má huáng* (Herba Ephedrae) has anti-allergic functions. Water and alcohol extracts can control eosinophil and mast cells that release histamine and other allergic chemicals. *Mǔ lì* (Concha Ostreae) contains calcium. This calcium has anti-allergic effects and can stop itching. There is a synergistic relationship between these two drugs. In the clinic, *má huáng* (Herba Ephedrae) 3-6g is used in combination with *mǔ lì* (Concha Ostreae) 30g (decocted first) to treat wind-cold and cold type of chronic urticaria.

2) *Zǐ sū yè* **(Folium Perillae) and** *fáng fēng* **(Radix Saposhnikoviae) to treat Stomach and Intestine acute urticaria:**

Zǐ sū yè (Folium Perillae) is pungent and slightly dry in flavor, warm in property, and has the functions of coursing wind, expelling the exterior and scattering cold, moving qi to remove stagnation from Spleen and Stomach, removing the toxicity of fish and crab, and improving the function of the gastrointestinal system. *Fáng fēng* (Radix Saposhnikoviae) is pungent and sweet in flavor, slightly warm in property, not dry but moistening, can both float and ascend, and is a marvelous herb to dispel wind. It has the functions of dispelling wind, releasing the exterior and stopping itching. The combination of these two herbs can strengthen the expelling action. For those allergic to fish and crab (which is thought to be caused by the toxins of fish and crabs), *zǐ sū yè* (Folium Perillae) can be added to remove the toxicity. Modern pharmacological studies showed that a water extract of *zǐ sū yè* (Folium Perillae) had middling restraining effect on mast cells releasing histamine, when mast cells induced by Con A substances and compound 48/80. Giving rats *Fang Feng Jian* can enhance peritoneal macrophage phagocytosis. The combination of these two herbs can enhance immune function and anti-allergic effects. Clinically, *zǐ sū yè* (Folium Perillae) 15g and *fáng fēng* (Radix Saposhnikoviae) 15g are often used to treat acute gastroenteritis urticaria caused by allergies to seafood and fish.

3) *Yú xīng cǎo* **(Herba Houttuyniae) and** *bái xiān pí* **(Cortex Dictamni) to treat damp-heat acute urticaria:**

Yú xīng cǎo (Herba Houttuyniae) has the functions of clearing heat and resolving toxin, draining dampness and inducing urination. *Bái xiān pí* (Cortex Dictamni) has the functions of clearing heat and resolving toxin, draining dampness and relieving itching. *Yú xīng cǎo* (Herba Houttuyniae) enters the Lung meridian and discharges through urination. *Bái xiān pí* (Cortex Dictamni) enters the Spleen and Stomach meridians and clears damp-heat from the gastrointestinal system. The combination of these two herbs can work together in the upper and lower parts of the body so as to dispel wind, resolve dampness and relieve itching. Modern pharmacological studies showed that the volatile oil of *yú xīng cǎo* (Herba Houttuyniae) has a significant anti-allergic effect. The volatile oil of *yú xīng cǎo* (Herba Houttuyniae) can significantly antagonize contractions of guinea pig ileum that has been induced by histamine and acetylcholine. Clinically, *yú xīng cǎo* (Herba Houttuyniae) 20-30g and *bái xiān pí* (Cortex Dictamni) 15g can be used to treat internal damp-heat urticaria.

4) *Xú cháng qīng* (Radix et Rhizoma Cynanchi Paniculati) and *mǔ dān pí* (Cortex Moutan) to treat acute and chronic blood heat (blood stagnation) urticaria:

Xú cháng qīng (Radix et Rhizoma Cynanchi Paniculati) has the functions of dispelling wind and relieving itching, and activating blood circulation. *Mǔ dān pí* (Cortex Moutan) has the functions of clearing heat and cooling blood, moving blood and removing blood stasis. The combination of these two herbs can strengthen the functions of moving blood, dispelling wind and relieving itching. Modern pharmacological research shows that both *xú cháng qīng* (Radix et Rhizoma Cynanchi Paniculati) and *mǔ dān pí* (Cortex Moutan) contain paeonol. Paeonol has a marked restraining function in cases of Ⅰ, Ⅲ, and Ⅳ type allergies. It does not affect the formation of specific antibodies, but can selectively inhibit the hemolytic process of complement classical pathway and regulate immune function. In clinic, *xú cháng qīng* (Radix et Rhizoma Cynanchi Paniculati) 15g and *mǔ dān pí* (Cortex Moutan) 10-15g can be used to treat blood heat and blood stasis urticaria.

5) *Wū méi* (Fructus Mume) and *wǔ wèi zǐ* (Fructus Schisandrae Chinensis) to treat stubborn urticaria with yin deficiency and exuberant fire:

Wū méi (Fructus Mume) encourages the production of body fluids so as to stop thirst, and astringes the Intestines so as to stop diarrhea. It has the functions of clearing the upper, warming the lower, and astringing yin. It also has the function of expelling roundworms. *Wǔ wèi zǐ* (Fructus Schisandrae Chinensis) is warm but not dry in property, sourly astringing, bitterly heat clearing and saltily nourishing yin. It has the functions of astringing the Lung and nourishing yin, encouraging production of body fluids and stopping sweating, and calming the spirit and mind.

Wū méi (Fructus Mume) enters the Liver, Spleen and Large intestine channels and goes to the Lower Jiao. *Wǔ wèi zǐ* (Fructus Schisandrae Chinensis) enters the Heart channel. The combination of these two herbs can strengthen the function of astringing yin in the upper and lower. In clinic, *wū méi* (Fructus Mume) 15-20g and *wǔ wèi zǐ* (Fructus Schisandrae Chinensis) 10g are often used to treat stubborn urticaria from yin deficiency with exuberant fire, accompanied by severe pruritus and roundworm urticaria.

These herbs should be used based on pattern differentiations.

Summary

Urticaria is a commonly-encountered skin disease. Through long-term clinical practice, it has been recognized that in general, the etiologies of acute urticaria are easily found. After eliminating the causes, the urticaria easily disappears. For mild urticaria, the use of either Chinese medicine or biomedicine can achieve good results. But for sudden onset severe urticaria, laryngeal edema and anaphylactic shock can occur, and this should be treated with a combination of Chinese medicine and biomedicine. Hormone therapy or tracheotomy should be used in a timely fashion in order to save lives. But for those who have been treated with hormone therapy it is easy to have repeated reoccurrences with a transformation of the illness into chronic urticaria. The combination of

Chinese medicine and biomedicine can reduce rebound and recurrence rates from hormone withdrawal, and can improve the clinical treatment effect and shorten the duration of illness. In acute stage, hormones associated with Chinese medicine can be used. Herbs which have the functions of releasing the exterior by pungent flavor and cool property, clearing heat and cooling blood, clearing heat and relaxing bowels to remove food stagnation can be chosen according to pattern differentiation. After the symptoms are relieved, Chinese medicine can be used for another 2-3 weeks.

Chinese medicine is obviously good at preventing and reducing the reoccurrence of urticaria. Urticaria is caused by complicated factors and easily repeatedly reoccurs. The pathogenesis is related with decreased immunity. Chinese medicine can improve immunity so as to reduce the reoccurrence of urticaria. Therefore the combination of Chinese medicine and biomedicine is commonly used for chronic urticaria that is characterized by repeated reoccurrences. In the acute stage, a combination of Chinese medicine and biomedicine can be used. When the symptoms are relieved, the biomedicine can be reduced gradually until it is totally stopped. Chinese medicine can be used for another 1-2 months until the disease is completely stable. The combination of Chinese medicine and biomedicine can relieve symptoms quickly and reduce the recurrence rate of urticaria.

At the present time, the combination of Chinese medicine and biomedicine has produced encouraging results in the treatment of urticaria. However, there are still some questions which deserve our consideration: the key question is how to choose the best time to intervene with Chinese medicine according to the rule of basing treatments on pattern differentiation. There are studies that show promise of combining Chinese medicine with biomedicine. Therefore, in the future, we should gather all kinds of tools, effective treatments and drugs, to set up reliably effective therapies of combined Chinese medicine and biomedicine in order to prevent and cure acute and chronic urticaria. There should be technical specifications and evaluation criteria to explore effective ways of establishing a comprehensive evaluation of Chinese medicine and biomedicine treatment of acute and chronic urticaria. The use of evidence-based medicine and clinical epidemiology research methods can be used for verification and evaluation, so that there will be widely accepted methods of prevention and cure.

SELECTED QUOTES FROM CLASSICAL TEXTS

Discussion of the Origins of the Symptoms of Disease-Category of Wind Insidious Urticaria (诸病源侯论 · 风瘙隐疹候, *Zhū Bìng Yuán Hóu Lùn - Fēng Sào Yǐn Zhěn Hòu)* "Evils accumulated in the skin with wind-cold attack can cause wind insidious urticaria."

（《诸病源侯论 · 风瘙隐疹候》"邪气客于皮肤复逢风寒相折，则起风瘙隐疹。"）

Discussion of the Origins of the Symptoms of Disease-Category of Wind Pattern (诸病源侯论 · 风痦瘟候, *Zhū Bìng Yuán Hóu Lùn - Fēng Pēi Lěi Hóu)*" For patients with yang deficiency leading to profuse sweating, when the sweat is exposed to wind, the wind evil fights against the heat and causes urticaria."

（《诸病源侯论 · 风痦瘟候》"夫人阳气外虚则多汗，汗出当风，风气搏于肌肉，与热气并，则生痦瘟，状如麻豆甚者渐大。"）

The Essentials of The Golden Cabinet-Treatment Based on Pulse and Syndrome of Water Qi Evil (金匮要略 · 水气病邪脉证并治, *Jīn Guì Yào Lüè - Shuǐ Qì Bìng Xié Mài Zhèng Bìng Zhì)* "When wind evil attacks the body, it can manifest as insidious rashes with pruritus. The prutitus is caused by wind. After a long time it can be transformed into scabs."

(《金匮要略·水气病邪脉证并治》"风气相搏，风强则为隐疹，身体为痒，痒为泄风，久为痂癞")

Indispensable Tools for Pattern Treatment-Category of Wind Evil (证治准绳 · 风 门 , *Zhèng Zhì Zhǔn Shéng - Fēng Mén)* "Heat evil accumulated in the skin with wind-cold attack can cause insidious rashes. With more heat the color of the rashes is red; for more severe wind the color is white with pruritus or pain and can transform into sores if scratched."

(《证治准绳·风门》"夫邪客热在于皮肤，遇风寒所伤则起瘾疹，热多则色赤，风多则色白，甚者痒痛，搔之则成疮。)

Comprehensive Records of External Medicine-Category of Insidious Rashes (外科大成 · 瘾疹 , *Wài Kē Dà Chéng - Yǐn Zhěn)* "As for urticaria, small sized on the skin, averse to cold with a fever and whole-body pruritis. The classics say that if there is sweating with wind, then acne occurs. If heat is slight then the color is red, if heat is severe then the color is black. From phlegm heat in the Lungs, treatment should clear the Lungs, descend the phlegm and resolve the exterior."

(《外科大成·瘾疹》"瘾疹者，声小粒魇于皮肤之中，憎寒发热遍身瘙痒。经方：劳汗当风，乃痤痱。热微色赤，热甚色黑。由痰热在肺，治宜清肺降痰解表。)

Golden Mirror of the Medical Tradition- Important Treatments of the Skin Disease (医宗金鉴 · 外科心法要诀 , *Yī Zōng Jīn Jiàn - Wài Kē Xīn Fǎ Yào Jué):* "This disease is also called ghost wind lump. It can be caused by sweating exposed to wind or sleeping in cold. Wind evil tends to attack people with deficient exteriors. First there is pruritus on the skin, then skin rashes occur and gather into patches. For pruritus aggravated in the daytime *Qín Jiāo Niú Bàng Tāng* (秦艽牛蒡汤) can be used. For pruritus aggravated at night *Dāng Guī Yǐn Zi* (当归饮子) can be added."

（《医宗金鉴·外科心法要诀》"此证俗名鬼风疙瘩，有汗出受风，或露卧来凉，风邪多中表虚之人。初起皮肤作痒，次发扁疙瘩，形如豆瓣，堆累成片。日痒甚，宜服秦艽牛蒡汤；夜痒重者，宜当归饮子服之。"）

MODERN RESEARCH

Clinical Research

1. PATTERN DIFFERENTIATION AND CORRESPONDING TREATMENT

(1) Xuan Guo-wei divided 93 cases of chronic urticaria into six types according to pattern differentiation. Among these, 53 cases were cured, 37 cases were improved and only 1 case showed no change.

1) *Wei qi* not consolidated.

Treatment should increase qi, consolidate the exterior, dispel wind and scatter cold.

Use modified *Yù Píng Fēng Săn*.

Ingredients:

黄芪	huáng qí	15g	Radix Astragali
白术	bái zhú	10g	Rhizoma Atractylodis Macrocephalae
防风	fáng fēng	10g	Radix Saposhnikoviae
炙麻黄	zhì má huáng	10g	Herba Ephedrae (processed)
蝉蜕	chán tuì	10g	Periostracum Cicadae
浮小麦	fú xiǎo mài	10g	Fructus Tritici Levis
甘草	gān cǎo	10g	Radix et Rhizoma Glycyrrhizae

2) Stomach and Intestines disharmony.

Treatment should regulate the Stomach and Intestines.

Use modified *Bǎo Hé Wán* (保和丸).

Ingredients:

山楂	shān zhā	30g	Fructus Crataegi
麦芽	mài yá	30g	Fructus Hordei Germinatus
神曲	shén qū	15g	Massa Medicata Fermentata
茯苓	fú líng	15g	Poria
绵茵陈	mián yīn chén	15g	Herba Artemisiae Scopariae
苏叶	sū yè	15g	Folium Perillae
黄芩	huáng qín	15g	Radix Scutellariae
枳实	zhǐ shí	12g	Fructus Aurantii Immaturus
白术	bái zhú	12g	Rhizoma Atractylodis Macrocephalae
法夏	fǎ xià	9g	Rhizoma Pinelliae Praeparatum
陈皮	chén pí	6g	Pericarpium Citri Reticulatae

3) Qi and blood stagnation.

Treatment should activate blood and remove blood stasis, regulate blood circulation, and dispel wind.

Use modified *Xuè Fǔ Zhú Yū Tāng* (血府逐瘀汤).

Ingredients:

生地	shēng dì	15g	Radix Rehmanniae Recens
赤芍	chì sháo	15g	Radix Paeoniae Rubra
桃仁	táo rén	15g	Semen Juglandis
秦艽	qín jiāo	15g	Radix Gentianae Macrophyllae
当归	dāng guī	10g	Radix Angelicae Sinensis
红花	hóng huā	10g	Flos Carthami
川芎	chuān xiōng	6g	Rhizoma Chuanxiong
地龙	dì lóng	12g	Pheretima
川蜈蚣（焙干研末冲服）	chuān wú gōng	2pieces	Scolopendra(fire dried, ground into powder, taken with water)
甘草	gān cǎo	9g	Radix et Rhizoma Glycyrrhizae
枳壳	zhǐ qiào	9g	Fructus Aurantii

4) Insufficiency of the Lung and Kidney.

Treatment should nourish the Lung and Kidney.

Use a modified *Liù Wèi Dì Huáng Tāng*.

Ingredients:

山萸肉	shān yú ròu	15g	Fructus Corni
淮山	huái shān	15g	Rhizoma Dioscoreae
茯苓	fú líng	15g	Poria
熟地	shú dì	15g	Radix Rehmanniae Praeparata
丹皮	dān pí	15g	Cortex Moutan
泽泻	zé xiè	15g	Rhizoma Alismatis
乌梅	wū méi	15g	Fructus Mume
首乌	shǒu wū	15g	Radix Polygoni Multiflori
白蒺藜	bái jí lí	15g	Fructus Tribuli
五味子	wǔ wèi zǐ	10g	Fructus Schisandrae Chinensis
甘草	*gān cǎo*	9g	Radix et Rhizoma Glycyrrhizae

5) Disharmony of *Chong* and *Ren* vessels.

Treatment should regulate the *Chong* and *Ren*.

Use a modified *Dān Zhī Xiāo Yáo Sǎn* (丹栀逍遥散).

Ingredients:

丹皮	dān pí	15g	Cortex Moutan
白芍	bái sháo	15g	Radix Paeoniae Alba
茯苓	fú líng	15g	Poria
夜交藤	yè jiāo téng	15g	Caulis Polygoni Multiflori
寮刁竹	liáo diāo zhú	15g	Herba et Radice Cynanchi Paniculati
当归	dāng guī	10g	Radix Angelicae Sinensis
白术	bái zhú	10g	Rhizoma Atractylodis Macrocephalae
柴胡	chái hú	10g	Radix Bupleuri
栀子	zhī zǐ	10g	Fructus Gardeniae
甘草	gān cǎo	10g	Radix et Rhizoma Glycyrrhizae

6) Deficiency of qi and blood.

Treatment should tonify qi and blood, and reinforce Heart and Spleen.

Use a modified *Dāng Guī Yǐn Zi*.

Ingredients:

生地	shēng dì	15g	Radix Rehmanniae Recens
白芍	bái sháo	15g	Radix Paeoniae Alba
首乌	shǒu wū	15g	Radix Polygoni Multiflori
白蒺藜	bái jí lí	15g	Fructus Tribuli
夜交藤	yè jiāo téng	15g	Caulis Polygoni Multiflori
当归	dāng guī	12g	Radix Angelicae Sinensis
防风	fáng fēng	12g	Radix Saposhnikoviae
黄芪	huáng qí	12g	Radix Astragali
白术	bái zhú	12g	Rhizoma Atractylodis Macrocephalae
乌梅	wū méi	12g	Fructus Mume
甘草	gān cǎo	10g	Radix et Rhizoma Glycyrrhizae
引芎	yǐn xiōng	9g	Rhizoma Chuanxiong

All of the formulas discussed above should be decocted with water and taken as 1 dose per day. 15 doses is a course of treatment [1 – 3].

(2) Zhou Bai-chuan always attaches importance to blood in his treatment of urticaria. He considers urticaria a deficiency pattern and he treats patients according to clinical pattern differentiation. [4]

1) Blood deficiency with wind attack.

Treatment should nourish blood and course wind.

Use a modified *Sì Wù Tāng* with *Má Huáng Lián Qiào Chì Xiǎo Dòu Sǎn* (麻黄连翘赤小豆散).

Ingredients：

生地	shēng dì	12g	Radix Rehmanniae Recens
当归	dāng guī	12g	Radix Angelicae Sinensis
川芎	chuān xiōng	9g	Rhizoma Chuanxiong
白芍	bái sháo	12g	Radix Paeoniae Alba
赤芍	chì sháo	12g	Radix Paeoniae Rubra
麻黄	má huáng	6g	Herba Ephedrae
连翘	lián qiào	12g	Fructus Forsythiae

赤小豆	chì xiǎo dòu	30g	Semen Phaseoli
防风	fáng fēng	9g	Radix Saposhnikoviae
黄芪	huáng qí	18g	Radix Astragali
杏仁	xìng rén	12g	Semen Armeniacae Amarum
甘草	gān cǎo	3g	Radix et Rhizoma Glycyrrhizae

2) Blood heat with wind attack.

Treatment should course wind and cool blood, clear heat and resolve toxin.

Use *Jīng Fáng Xiāo Fēng Sǎn* (荆防消风散).

Ingredients:

浮萍	fú píng	9g	Herba Spirodelae
荆芥	jīng jiè	18g	Herba Schizonepetae
生地	shēng dì	18g	Radix Rehmanniae Recens
丹皮	dān pí	12g	Cortex Moutan
赤芍	chì sháo	18g	Radix Paeoniae Rubra
紫金皮	zǐ jīn pí	30g	Cortex Arisiae Japonicae
金银花	jīn yín huā	15g	Flos Lonicerae Japonicae
连翘	lián qiào	15g	Fructus Forsythiae
蝉衣	chán yī	9g	Periostracum Cicadae
刺蒺藜	cì jí lí	30g	Fructus Tribuli

3) Disharmony between *ying* and *wei* with exterior deficiency.

Treatment should increase qi, consolidate the exterior, and regulate and harmonize the *ying* and *wei*.

Use a modified *Yù Píng Fēng Sǎn*.

Ingredients:

黄芪	huáng qí	30g	Radix Astragali
白术	bái zhú	12g	Rhizoma Atractylodis Macrocephalae
防风	fáng fēng	9g	Radix Saposhnikoviae
桂枝	guì zhī	9g	Ramulus Cinnamomi
白芍	bái sháo	12g	Radix Paeoniae Alba

炙甘草	zhì gān cǎo	6g	Radix et Rhizoma Glycyrrhizae
大枣	dà zǎo	12pieces	Fructus Jujubae
生姜	shēng jiāng	9g	Rhizoma Zingiberis Recens
当归	dāng guī	12g	Radix Angelicae Sinensis

4) Deficiency of the Middle Jiao with concurrent wind cold.

Treatment should warm the Middle Jiao, expel cold, ascend yang and resolve toxin.

Use a modified *Xiǎo Jiàn Zhōng Tāng* (小建中汤) with *Shēng Má Gé Gēn Tāng* (升麻葛根汤).

Ingredients:

黄芪	huáng qí	30g	Radix Astragali
桂枝	guì zhī	9g	Ramulus Cinnamomi
白芍	bái sháo	18g	Radix Paeoniae Alba
炙甘草	zhì gān cǎo	6g	Radix et Rhizoma Glycyrrhizae Praeparata
大枣	dà zǎo	12pieces	Fructus Jujubae
饴糖	yí táng	30g	Saccharum Granorum
当归	dāng guī	12g	Radix Angelicae Sinensis
升麻	shēng má	9g	Rhizoma Cimicifugae
葛根	gé gēn	12g	Radix Puerariae Lobatae

(3) Zhu Liang-chun believes that although there are numerous etiological factors and pathogeneses of urticaria, they all have a close relationship with both internal and external wind. The most important treatment should focus on dispelling wind. Zhu also knows how to handle insect herbs like *wū shāo shé* (Zaocys), and *jiāng cán* (Bombyx Batryticatus). [5]

1) Usually in the early stages wind heat stays in the *ying* aspect. During that time treatment should dispel wind, purge heat, and cool and activate blood.

Jiāng cán (Bombyx Batryticatus) is good for dispelling wind and purging heat and is effective for wind heat urticaria. Zhu has two effective formulas.

Formula 1:

僵蚕	jiāng cán	60g	Bombyx Batryticatus
蛇蜕	shé tuì	30g	Periostracum Serpentis
生大黄	shēng dà huáng	120g	Raw Radix et Rhizoma Rhei
广姜黄	guǎng jiāng huáng	45g	Rhizoma Curcumae Longae

Each kind of herb should be ground into a powder. Take 6g with sugar water once a day.

Formula 2:

僵蚕	jiāng cán	Bombyx Batryticatus
姜黄	jiāng huáng	Rhizoma Curcumae Longae
蝉衣	chán yī	Periostracum Cicadae
乌梢蛇	wū shāo shé	Zaocys

The herbs should be in equal amounts and then ground into a powder. 4-5 grams are taken each time.

The two decoctions have almost the same function. However, the former is more suitable for strong patients and the latter is more suitable for the patients with Spleen qi deficiency and severe wind heat.

2) Patients whom suffer from long-term *ying* deficiency should be treated by nourishing *ying*, activating blood, and dispelling wind.

If the patient suffers from long-term *ying* deficiency, the wind will fight with heat and there will be stagnation, causing a rash to appear everywhere on the skin. The patient will then suffer from unbearable itching, and possibly restlessness and insomnia. Treatment should take in account that long term disease causes blood stasis and deficiency. *Ying* deficiency is the cause of the disease; stagnated blood and enduring wind qi are the manifestations. Treatment should nourish *ying*, activate blood, and dispel wind.

Use a modified *Sì Wù Tāng*, *shēng dì* (Radix Rehmanniae Recens) should be in a large dose of 30g, it can be accompanied by:

益母草	yì mǔ cǎo	Herba Leonuri
紫草	zǐ cǎo	Radix Arnebiae
红花	hóng huā	Flos Carthami
白鲜皮	bái xiān pí	Cortex Dictamni
白蒺藜	bái jí lí	Fructus Tribuli
徐长卿	xú cháng qīng	Radix et Rhizoma Cynanchi Paniculati

(4) Zhang Zuo-zhou has accumulated much experience in treating urticaria. He specializes in making prescriptions. Zhang divides chronic urticaria into 4 patterns based on clinical manifestations. [6]

1) Exterior deficient and not consolidated, with disharmony between *ying* and *wei* :

Treatment should strengthen the wei and regulate *ying*. Assist the treatment by sourly constraining.

Use *Gù Wèi Yù Fēng Tāng*.

Ingredients:

北芪	běi qí	Radix Astragali
防风	fáng fēng	Radix Saposhnikoviae
白术	bái zhú	Rhizoma Atractylodis Macrocephalae
党参	dǎng shēn	Radix Codonopsis
桂枝	guì zhī	Ramulus Cinnamomi
白芍	bái sháo	Radix Paeoniae Alba
白鲜皮	bái xiān pí	Cortex Dictamni
秦艽	qín jiāo	Radix Gentianae Macrophyllae
白芥子	bái jiè zǐ	Semen Brassica alba
乌梅	wū méi	Fructus Mume
五味子	wǔ wèi zǐ	Fructus Schisandrae Chinensis

If there are heat symptoms then *bái jiè zǐ* (Semen Brassica alba) should be removed and *qīng hāo* (Herba Artemisiae Annuae) should be added.

If the patient sweats a lot, then *mǔ lì* (Concha Ostreae) should be added.

If the patient suffers from severe itching then *cì jí lí* (Fructus Tribuli) should be added.

2) Blood and qi deficiency generating internal wind:

Treatment should nourish blood and extinguish wind, treating both the internal and external patterns.

Use *Yǎng Xuè Xī Fēng Tāng* (养血熄风汤).

Ingredients:

当归	dāng guī	Radix Angelicae Sinensis
黄芪	huáng qí	Radix Astragali
何首乌	hé shǒu wū	Radix Polygoni Multiflori
白芍	bái sháo	Radix Paeoniae Alba
五味子	wǔ wèi zǐ	Fructus Schisandrae Chinensis
乌蛇	wū shé	Zaocys
全虫	quán chóng	Scorpio
白鲜皮	bái xiān pí	Cortex Dictamni
羌活	qiāng huó	Rhizoma et Radix Notopterygii

For a stubborn rash that does not lessen, add *wú gōng* (Scolopendra) (3 pieces).

For a dim rash, purple lips and a dark tongue, add *táo rén* (Semen Juglandis), *hóng huā* (Flos Carthami), and *guì zhī* (Ramulus Cinnamomi), so as to activate the blood and open the collaterals.

If the rash occurs while a woman has her period, then it is caused by blood deficiency and disharmony between the *Chong* and *Ren* vessels. In that case, add *yì mǔ cǎo* (Herba Leonuri) so as to nourish blood and regulate menstruation.

3) Yin deficiency and internal heat:

Treatment should nourish yin, clear heat, subdue yang, and extinguish wind.

Use *Yǎng Yīn Níng Qián Tāng* (养阴宁葶汤).

Ingredients:

生地	shēng dì	Radix Rehmanniae Recens
白芍	bái sháo	Radix Paeoniae Alba
女贞子	nǚ zhēn zǐ	Fructus Ligustri Lucidi
黄芪	huáng qí	Radix Astragali
五味子	wǔ wèi zǐ	Fructus Schisandrae Chinensis
地骨皮	dì gǔ pí	Cortex Lycii
丹皮	dān pí	Cortex Moutan
生牡蛎	shēng mǔ lì	Concha Ostreae
珍珠母	zhēn zhū mǔ	Concha Margaritifera
白鲜皮	bái xiān pí	Cortex Dictamni
秦艽	qín jiāo	Radix Gentianae Macrophyllae

For severe deficiency heat, add *huáng qín* (Radix Scutellariae), and *qīng hāo* (Herba Artemisiae Annuae).

For severe itching, add *chán yī* (Periostracum Cicadae).

4) Stomach and Intestine dampness and heat:

Treatment should clear heat, rectify the Spleen, and diffuse and transform damp turbidity.

Use modified *Píng Wèi Sǎn* (平胃散).

Ingredients:

苍术	cāng zhú	Rhizoma Atractylodis
厚朴	hòu pò	Cortex Magnoliae Officinalis
茯苓	fú líng	Poria
茵陈	yīn chén	Herba Artemisiae Scopariae
青蒿	qīng hāo	Herba Artemisiae Annuae
黄芩	huáng qín	Radix Scutellariae
藿香	huò xiāng	Herba Pogostemonis
佩兰	pèi lán	Herba Eupatorii
白鲜皮	bái xiān pí	Cortex Dictamni
刺蒺藜	cì jí lí	Fructus Tribuli

For constipation, add *jiāo bīng láng* (Semen Arecae processed).

(5) In order to treat urticaria, Gong Guo-mu-liang divides the disease into four patterns based on clinical manifestations. These patterns are wind-cold type, wind-heat type, Stomach and Intestines type, and blood deficiency type. [7]

1) Wind-heat type:

Treatment should dispel wind and clear heat.

Use modified *Xiāo Fēng Săn* (消风散).

Ingredients:

荆芥	jīng jiè	9g	Herba Schizonepetae
防风	fáng fēng	9g	Radix Saposhnikoviae
牛蒡子	niú bàng zĭ	9g	Fructus Arctii
蝉衣	chán yī	9g	Periostracum Cicadae
薄荷（后下）	bò hé	6g	Herba Menthae（decocted later）
知母	zhī mŭ	9g	Rhizoma Anemarrhenae
生地	shēng dì	15g	Radix Rehmanniae Recens
金银花	jīn yín huā	9g	Flos Lonicerae Japonicae
连翘	lián qiào	9g	Fructus Forsythiae
生石膏	shēng shí gāo	30g	Gypsum Fibrosum

2) Wind-cold type:

Treatment should dispel wind and scatter cold.

Use modified *Guì Zhī Má Huáng Gè Bàn Tāng*.

Ingredients:

桂枝	guì zhī	9g	Ramulus Cinnamomi
麻黄	má huáng	9g	Herba Ephedrae
白芍	bái sháo	9g	Radix Paeoniae Alba
甘草	gān căo	9g	Radix et Rhizoma Glycyrrhizae
浮萍	fú píng	9g	Herba Spirodelae
苏叶	sū yè	9g	Folium Perillae
防风	fáng fēng	9g	Radix Saposhnikoviae
生姜	shēng jiāng	9g	Rhizoma Zingiberis Recens

3) Stomach and Intestine type:

Treatment should dispel wind and resolve the exterior, open the *fu* organs and drain heat.

Prescription:

荆芥	jīng jiè	9g	Herba Schizonepetae
防风	fáng fēng	9g	Radix Saposhnikoviae
茵陈	yīn chén	15g	Herba Artemisiae Scopariae
制大黄	zhì dà huáng	9g	Radix et Rhizoma Rhei processed
生山楂	shēng shān zhā	6g	Raw Fructus Crataegi
苍术	cāng zhú	9g	Rhizoma Atractylodis
苦参	kǔ shēn	9g	Radix Sophorae Flavescentis
生甘草	shēng gān cǎo	9g	Raw Radix et Rhizoma Glycyrrhizae

4) Blood deficiency type:

Treatment should nourish blood and dispel wind.

Use modified *Sì Wù Tāng*.

Ingredients:

当归	dāng guī	9g	Radix Angelicae Sinensis
熟地	shú dì	15g	Radix Rehmanniae Praeparata
白芍	bái sháo	9g	Radix Paeoniae Alba
川芎	chuān xiōng	9g	Rhizoma Chuanxiong
首乌	shǒu wū	15g	Radix Polygoni Multiflori
荆芥	jīng jiè	9g	Herba Schizonepetae
防风	fáng fēng	9g	Radix Saposhnikoviae
豨莶草	xī xiān cǎo	15g	Herba Siegesbeckiae

(6) In Professor. Wang Yu-xi's opinion, urticaria has complicated etiological factors. During the acute stage, the patterns are usually exterior and excess. Treatment should dispel wind, clear heat, scatter cold, cool blood, and resolve toxin. During the chronic stage, the patterns usually have dampness, deficiency and blood stasis. Treatment should eliminate dampness, tonify deficiency, activate blood, and transform blood stasis.

1) The early stage of the wind-cold type is caused by external wind-cold attack, and disharmony between *ying* and *wei*.

Long-term disease will cause the exterior to become deficient and the wei to become unconsolidated. Thus it becomes easy to be attacked by wind-cold evil. This manifests as light red skin rashes, especially on exposed areas such as the head, face, feet and hands. This condition is aggravated by wind or cold, and is relieved by warmth. The tongue is pale, with a thin white coat. There is a floating, tight or deep, moderate pulse. This is mainly cold urticaria and should be treated by dispelling wind and expelling cold, and regulating *ying* and *wei*.

Use a modified *Má Huáng Guì Zhī Gè Bàn Tāng*, *Yù Píng Fēng Sǎn* and *Guì Zhī Tāng*.

Ingredients:

黄芪	huáng qí	Radix Astragali
防风	fáng fēng	Radix Saposhnikoviae
白术	bái zhú	Rhizoma Atractylodis Macrocephalae
白芍	bái sháo	Radix Paeoniae Alba
桂枝	guì zhī	Ramulus Cinnamomi
杏仁	xìng rén	Semen Armeniacae Amarum
荆芥	jīng jiè	Herba Schizonepetae
麻黄	má huáng	Herba Ephedrae
蝉衣	chán yī	Periostracum Cicadae
白鲜皮	bái xiān pí	Cortex Dictamni
甘草	gān cǎo	Radix et Rhizoma Glycyrrhizae
生姜	shēng jiāng	Rhizoma Zingiberis Recens
大枣	dà zǎo	Fructus Jujubae

2) The wind-heat pattern is caused by wind-heat first accumulating on the surface of the body and damaging *ying* and blood, causing a disharmony between *ying* and *wei*.

After a long time, wind-heat evil depresses in the muscles, and this leads to the inability of the exterior to outthrust and the interior to course and drain. This manifests as red skin rashes that are aggravated by heat and relieved by cold. They occur mainly on the upper body, and are accompanied by a sore and swollen throat, a floating, slippery and rapid pulse, a red tongue body, and a thin-white or yellow coat. This should be treated by dispelling wind and clearing heat.

Use a modified *Shū Fēng Qīng Rè Yǐn*.

Ingredients:

荆芥	jīng jiè	Herba Schizonepetae
防风	fáng fēng	Radix Saposhnikoviae
牛蒡子	niú bàng zǐ	Fructus Arctii
白蒺藜	bái jí lí	Fructus Tribuli
蝉衣	chán yī	Periostracum Cicadae
生地黄	shēng dì huáng	Radix Rehmanniae Recens
丹参	dān shēn	Radix et Rhizoma Salviae Miltiorrhizae
赤芍	chì sháo	Radix Paeoniae Rubra
炒山栀	chǎo shān zhī	Fructus Gardeniae stir fried
黄芩	huáng qín	Radix Scutellariae
银花	yín huā	Flos Lonicerae Japonicae
连翘	lián qiào	Fructus Forsythiae
生甘草	shēng gān cǎo	Radix et Rhizoma Glycyrrhizae

3) The disharmony between *Chong* and *Ren* type is caused by deficiency of Liver and Kidney, disharmony between *Chong* and *Ren*, and malnourishment of the skin engendering wind and dryness accumulating on the skin.

This occurs mainly during menstruation or pregnancy and labor. The skin rashes occur 2-3 days before menstruation, and disappear after menstruation. They are distributed mainly on the lower abdomen, lumbar-sacral region and thighs. The tongue body is light red, with a thin-white or scanty coat. The pulse is wiry-thin or wiry-slippery. The treatment principle should be to regulate the *Chong* and *Ren*.

Use a modified *Sì Wù Tāng* with *Er Xiān Tāng*.

Ingredients:

当归	dāng guī	Radix Angelicae Sinensis
赤芍	chì sháo	Radix Paeoniae Rubra

川芎	chuān xiōng	Rhizoma Chuanxiong
生地黄	shēng dì huáng	Radix Rehmanniae Recens
川牛膝	chuān niú xī	Radix Achyranthis Bidentatae
丹参	dān shēn	Radix et Rhizoma Salviae Miltiorrhizae
益母草	yì mǔ cǎo	Herba Leonuri
黄柏	huáng bǎi	Cortex Phellodendri Chinensis
仙茅	xiān máo	Rhizoma Curculiginis
仙灵脾	xiān líng pí	Epimedium brevicornum Maxim
巴戟天	bā jǐ tiān	Radix Morindae Officinalis
淫羊藿	yín yáng huò	Herba Epimedii

4) The damp-heat type is caused by internal dampness with external evil attacking.

It manifests as bright red skin rashes with lingering pruritus, abdominal pain, diarrhea, nausea, a red tongue body, a yellow-greasy coat, and a rapid or soggy-rapid pulse. The treatment principle should be to clear heat and drain dampness, dispel wind and relieve pain.

Use a modified *Cán Shā Yǐn* (蚕砂饮).

Ingredients:

蚕砂	cán shā	Faeces Bombycis
蚤休	zǎo xiū	Rhizoma Paridis
丹参	dān shēn	Radix et Rhizoma Salviae Miltiorrhizae
白鲜皮	bái xiān pí	Cortex Dictamni
地肤子	dì fū zǐ	Fructus Kochiae
蛇床子	shé chuáng zǐ	Fructus Cnidii
蝉蜕	chán tuì	Periostracum Cicadae
槐花	huái huā	Flos Sophorae
牡丹皮	mǔ dān pí	Cortex Moutan
赤芍	chì sháo	Radix Paeoniae Rubra
生甘草	shēng gān cǎo	Radix et Rhizoma Glycyrrhizae

5) The blood-heat type with fire in the Heart channel is caused by heat in the blood level engendering wind.

It manifests with symptoms that are worse at night. First there are burning, stabbing, and itching sensations on the skin. Then more and more rashes occur as the patient scratches the skin. This is accompanied by vexation, dry mouth with a desire for fluids, a red tongue body, a scanty coat, and a wiry, slippery and rapid pulse. This is usually seen in artificial urticaria, also called dermographic disease. The treatment principle should be to cool blood, clear heat, dispel wind and stop itching.

Use modified *Xiāo Fēng Sǎn*.

Ingredients:

荆芥	jīng jiè	Herba Schizonepetae
防风	fáng fēng	Radix Saposhnikoviae
生地黄	shēng dì huáng	Radix Rehmanniae Recens
当归	dāng guī	Radix Angelicae Sinensis
蝉蜕	chán tuì	Periostracum Cicadae
苦参	kǔ shēn	Radix Sophorae Flavescentis
白蒺藜	bái jí lí	Fructus Tribuli
知母	zhī mǔ	Rhizoma Anemarrhenae
生石膏	shēng shí gāo	Gypsum Fibrosum
生甘草	shēng gān cǎo	Radix et Rhizoma Glycyrrhizae

6) The blood stasis type is caused by blood stasis obstructing the channels, the *ying* and *wei qi* not diffusing and wind-cold or wind-heat mutually contending.

This manifests as dark red skin rashes, a murky gray complexion, purple lips, and wheals that occur easily on areas of the body that are pressed by a waistband or watchband (stress urticaria). The tongue body is purple with petechia, and the pulse is thin and choppy. This should be treated by invigorating blood, dispelling wind, transforming blood stasis, and stopping itching.

Use modified *Táo Hóng Sì Wù Tāng*.

Ingredients:

桃仁	táo rén	Semen Juglandis
红花	hóng huā	Flos Carthami
地龙	dì lóng	Pheretima
皂刺	zào cì	Spina Gleditsiae
当归	dāng guī	Radix Angelicae Sinensis
川芎	chuān xiōng	Rhizoma Chuanxiong
赤芍	chì sháo	Radix Paeoniae Rubra
鬼箭羽	guǐ jiàn yǔ	Euonymi Lignum Suberalatum
丹参	dān shēn	Radix et Rhizoma Salviae Miltiorrhizae
蝉蜕	chán tuì	Periostracum Cicadae

For skin rashes on the upper limbs, add *sāng zhī* (Ramulus Mori) and *guì zhī* (Ramulus Cinnamomi).

For skin rashes on the lower limbs, add *chuān niú xī* (Radix Achyranthis Bidentatae).

7) The blood deficiency type is caused by Liver losing nourishment, thus engendering internal wind.

This pattern belongs to the blood deficiency engendering wind category. It occurs mainly in the elderly or after a long-term disease. There are light red skin rashes that are alleviated in the daytime and aggravated at night or with fatigue. The tongue is pale with a thin coat. There is a wiry and thready pulse. This should be treated by nourishing blood, invigorating blood, dispelling wind, and stopping itching.

Use modified *Dāng Guī Yǐn Zi.*

Ingredients:

当归	dāng guī	Radix Angelicae Sinensis
白芍	bái sháo	Radix Paeoniae Alba

川芎	chuān xiōng	Rhizoma Chuanxiong
生地	shēng dì	Radix Rehmanniae Recens
白蒺藜	bái jí lí	Fructus Tribuli
荆芥穗	jīng jiè suì	Spica Schizonepetae
防风	fáng fēng	Radix Saposhnikoviae
何首乌	hé shǒu wū	Radix Polygoni Multiflori
黄芪	huáng qí	Radix Astragali
炙甘草	zhì gān cǎo	Radix et Rhizoma Glycyrrhizae Praeparata

For exuberant wind, add *jiāng cán* (Bombyx Batryticatus), *wū shāo shé* (Zaocys), and *quán xiē* (Scorpio).

For exuberant heat, add *chán tuì* (Periostracum Cicadae) and *bò hé* (Herba Menthae).

8) Non-consolidation of the exterior is caused by sweating exposed to wind or sleeping in the cold.

As for profuse sweating, it is mainly caused by deficient yang qi, *wei* not consolidated, and a disharmony between *ying* and *wei* causing sluggish qi and blood circulation and malnourishment of the skin. This should be treated by warming yang, tonifying qi, consolidating the exterior, and resisting wind.

Use modified *Yù Píng Fēng Sǎn* with *Guì Zhī Tāng*.

Ingredients:

桂枝	guì zhī	Ramulus Cinnamomi
白芍	bái sháo	Radix Paeoniae Alba
生姜	shēng jiāng	Rhizoma Zingiberis Recens
大枣	dà zǎo	Fructus Jujubae
黄芪	huáng qí	Radix Astragali
防风	fáng fēng	Radix Saposhnikoviae
白术	bái zhú	Rhizoma Atractylodis Macrocephalae
茯苓	fú líng	Poria
甘草	gān cǎo	Radix et Rhizoma Glycyrrhizae

For aversion to wind, use *Guì Zhī Jiā Fù Zǐ Tāng* (桂枝加附子汤)[8].

(7) Professor Shi Guan-qing believes that urticaria can be divided into three patterns based on symptoms. These are damp heat accumulating in the lungs with a loss of diffusion and draining, Spleen and Stomach not transporting with wind damp evil stagnation, and disharmony of *ying* and *wei* with wind evil sneak-attacking.

1) The damp-heat retention in the Lungs with a loss of diffusion and draining type.

It is caused mainly by sweat exposed to wind, damp-heat accumulating in the Lungs, a loss of diffusion and draining and evil lodging in the skin and flesh. This is induced by external damp-heat in the summer and should be treated with *Má Huáng Lián Qiào Chì Xiǎo Dòu Tāng*. This prescription originated from Zhang Zhong-jin's treatment of yang jaundice caused by internal accumulation of cold, dampness and heat with the exterior symptoms. According to the theory that the "Lung controls the skin", this formula can be used to treat urticaria caused by damp-heat retention in the Lung leading to a loss of diffusion and draining. This prescription has the functions of scattering wind-heat, diffusing Lung qi, and dispelling dampness. It can be modified with *dì fū zǐ* (Fructus Kochiae) and *bái xiān pí* (Cortex Dictamni) to dispel wind so as to stop itching. For eczema on the neck and chest that emerges and disappears with small blisters that exudate yellow fluids when scratched, treatment should clear heat, resolve toxin and dispel dampness. Using this formula as a treatment has good results.

2) The Spleen and Stomach not transporting with wind-damp depression and stagnation type.

It is caused by a failure of the Spleen to transport, with an external wind evil attack, leading to sluggish qi flow, induced by improper diet. Improper diet obstructs the Middle Jiao and depresses in the Spleen and Stomach, leading to severe abdominal pain, nausea, and diarrhea. The

Spleen governs the muscles, and so when the body surface is attacked by wind evil, it can manifest as insidious wind rashes. *Cāng zhú* (Rhizoma Atractylodis), *chén pí* （Pericarpium Citri Reticulatae） and *hòu pò* (Cortex Magnoliae Officinalis) can strengthen the Spleen and resolve dampness, dispel wind and stop itching. *Jīng jiè* (Herba Schizonepetae) and *fáng fēng* (Radix Saposhnikoviae) can diffuse and open the interstitial spaces, smooth the qi dynamic, and move the *ying* and *wei*. *Xú cháng qīng* (Radix et Rhizoma Cynanchi Paniculati) can not only dispel wind but also calm the mind and relieve itching. Indigestion is one of the important causative factors for this disease so promoting digestion to remove stagnation should be used to assist with strengthening the Spleen and draining dampness, dispelling wind and stopping itching. *Shān zhā* (Fructus Crataegi) and *shén qū* (Massa Medicata Fermentata) can strengthen the treatment effect.

3) The disharmony between *ying* and *wei* with wind evil attacking type.

It mainly manifests with a lingering course of disease without cure. It is caused by qi and blood deficiency, disharmony between yin and yang, *ying* and *wei*, *wei* not consolidated, and wind evil attacking. This should be treated by harmonizing *ying* and *wei*, dispelling wind and stopping itching. *Guì Zhī Jiā Lóng Gǔ Mǔ Lì Tāng* (桂枝加龙骨牡蛎汤) can be used to regulate *ying* and *wei*, and subdue yang into yin. This is also caused by external wind attack leading to wind-heat accumulation. Therefore *Xiǎo Chái Hú Tāng* (小柴胡汤) can course and scatter the wind heat evil, causing the qi dynamic of the whole body to be regulated. *Dì fū zǐ* (Fructus Kochiae) and *bái xiān pí* (Cortex Dictamni) can be used to dispel wind and stop itching. The combination of all of these herbs can regulate yin and yang, *ying* and *wei*, and exterior and interior so as to extinguish internal wind and cure the disease[9].

2. SPECIFIC FORMULAS

1) *Wū Shé Chán Tuì Tāng* (乌蛇蝉蜕汤)

乌梅	wū méi	20g	Fructus Mume
蝉蜕	chán tuì	12g	Periostracum Cicadae
蛇蜕	shé tuì	5g	Periostracum Serpentis
桂枝	guì zhī	10g	Ramulus Cinnamomi
白芍	bái sháo	10g	Radix Paeoniae Alba
生姜	shēng jiāng	3g	Rhizoma Zingiberis Recens
大枣	dà zǎo	6pieces	Fructus Jujubae

It was used to treat 46 cases of urticaria with a total effectiveness rate of 95.8%.[10]

2) *Qū Qián Tāng* (祛荨汤)

荆芥	jīng jiè	10g	Herba Schizonepetae
防风	fáng fēng	10g	Radix Saposhnikoviae
生地	shēng dì	15g	Radix Rehmanniae Recens
丹皮	dān pí	10g	Cortex Moutan
赤芍	chì sháo	10g	Radix Paeoniae Rubra
金银花	jīn yín huā	20g	Flos Lonicerae Japonicae
连翘	lián qiào	10g	Fructus Forsythiae
白鲜皮	bái xiān pí	12g	Cortex Dictamni
白蒺藜	bái jí lí	12g	Fructus Tribuli
蝉衣	chán yī	9g	Periostracum Cicadae
夜交藤	yè jiāo téng	20g	Caulis Polygoni Multiflori
炒枣仁	chǎo zǎo rén	15g	Semen Ziziphi Spinosae stir-fried
甘草	gān cǎo	6g	Radix et Rhizoma Glycyrrhizae

It was used to treat 60 cases of acute wind –heat pattern urticaria with a total effectiveness rate of 98.3%.[11]

3) *Gù Biǎo Qū Fēng Tāng* (固表祛风汤)

黄芪	huáng qí	30g	Radix Astragali
白术	bái zhú	20g	Rhizoma Atractylodis Macrocephalae

云苓	yún líng	15g	Poria
当归	dāng guī	15g	Radix Angelicae Sinensis
地肤子	dì fū zǐ	10g	Fructus Kochiae
蛇床子	shé chuáng zǐ	10g	Fructus Cnidii
防风	fáng fēng	9g	Radix Saposhnikoviae
生姜	shēng jiāng	12g	Rhizoma Zingiberis Recens
大枣	dà zǎo	5pieces	Fructus Jujubae

It was used to treat 16 cases of urticaria with all of the cases receiving good effects. [12]

4) *Kè Yǎng Tāng* （克痒汤）

公英	gōng yīng	15g	Herba Taraxaci
地丁	dì dīng	10g	Herba Violae
荆芥	jīng jiè	10g	Herba Schizonepetae
防风	fáng fēng	10g	Radix Saposhnikoviae
川芎	chuān xiōng	10g	Rhizoma Chuanxiong
白鲜皮	bái xiān pí	15g	Cortex Dictamni
地肤子	dì fū zǐ	10g	Fructus Kochiae
当归	dāng guī	10g	Radix Angelicae Sinensis
赤芍	chì sháo	10g	Radix Paeoniae Rubra
大黄	dà huáng	5g	Radix et Rhizoma Rhei
甘草	gān cǎo	3g	Radix et Rhizoma Glycyrrhizae

It was used to treat 39 cases of acute urticaria and 33 cases of chronic urticaria with a total effectiveness rate of 98.6%. [13]

5) *Jīng Fáng Sì Wù Tāng* （荆防四物汤）

荆芥	jīng jiè	10g	Herba Schizonepetae
防风	fáng fēng	10g	Radix Saposhnikoviae
当归	dāng guī	10g	Radix Angelicae Sinensis
川芎	chuān xiōng	10g	Rhizoma Chuanxiong
丹皮	dān pí	10g	Cortex Moutan
栀子	zhī zǐ	10g	Fructus Gardeniae
浮萍	fú píng	10g	Herba Spirodelae

生地	shēng dì	15g	Radix Rehmanniae Recens
赤芍	chì sháo	15g	Radix Paeoniae Rubra
地肤子	dì fū zǐ	15g	Fructus Kochiae
白鲜皮	bái xiān pí	15g	Cortex Dictamni
生首乌	shēng shǒu wū	15g	Raw Radix Polygoni Multiflori
胡麻仁	hú má rén	15g	Fructus Cannabis

It was used to treat 178 cases of urticaria with a total effectiveness rate of 99.3%. [14]

6) Huó Xuè Qū Fēng Tāng（活血祛风汤）

当归	dāng guī	12g	Radix Angelicae Sinensis
鸡血藤	jī xuè téng	12g	Caulis Spatholobi
生地	shēng dì	18g	Radix Rehmanniae Recens
丹参	dān shēn	10g	Radix et Rhizoma Salviae Miltiorrhizae
荆芥	jīng jiè	10g	Herba Schizonepetae
防风	fáng fēng	10g	Radix Saposhnikoviae
蝉衣	chán yī	6g	Periostracum Cicadae
浮萍	fú píng	9g	Herba Spirodelae
神曲	shén qū	9g	Massa Medicata Fermentata
甘草	gān cǎo	3g	Radix et Rhizoma Glycyrrhizae

Modification is made according to pattern differentiation.

For excessive wind, add *sāng yè* (Folium Mori), *bái jí lí* (Fructus Tribuli), and *jiāng cán* (Bombyx Batryticatus).

For severe heat, add *dān pí* (Cortex Moutan) and *dì dīng* (Herba Violae).

For severe dampness, add *cāng zhú* (Rhizoma Atractylodis), *zé xiè* (Rhizoma Alismatis), and *fú líng* (Poria).

For yin deficiency, add *dì gǔ pí* (Cortex Lycii), *mài dōng* (Radix Ophiopogonis), and *yù zhú* (Rhizoma Polygonati Odorati).

For wei qi not consolidated, add *huáng qí* (Radix Astragali).

The herbs should be decocted twice with water and taken twice a day, in the morning and in the evening. The treatment effect of chronic urticaria is marked. [15]

7) *Tuō Mǐn Tāng* （脱敏汤）

荆芥	jīng jiè	10g	Herba Schizonepetae
防风	fáng fēng	10g	Radix Saposhnikoviae
鸡血藤	jī xuè téng	20g	Caulis Spatholobi
茜草	qiàn cǎo	10g	Radix et Rhizoma Rubiae
紫草	zǐ cǎo	10g	Radix Arnebiae
旱莲草	hàn lián cǎo	10g	Herba Ecliptae
桂枝	guì zhī	6g	Ramulus Cinnamomi
白芍	bái sháo	10g	Radix Paeoniae Alba
甘草	gān cǎo	6g	Radix et Rhizoma Glycyrrhizae

It was used to treat 46 cases of stubborn urticaria with a total effectiveness rate of 97.8%. [16]

8) *Xiāo Zhěn Yǐn* （消疹饮）

麻黄	má huáng	10g	Herba Ephedrae
当归	dāng guī	12g	Radix Angelicae Sinensis
防风	fáng fēng	12g	Radix Saposhnikoviae
黄芩	huáng qín	12g	Radix Scutellariae
甘草	gān cǎo	12g	Radix et Rhizoma Glycyrrhizae
乌梢蛇	wū shāo shé	10g	Zaocys
地肤子	dì fū zǐ	10g	Fructus Kochiae
荆芥	jīng jiè	10g	Herba Schizonepetae
丹皮	dān pí	10g	Cortex Moutan
白芍	bái sháo	10g	Radix Paeoniae Alba
刺蒺藜	cì jí lí	18g	Fructus Tribuli
生地	shēng dì	18g	Radix Rehmanniae Recens
玄参	xuán shēn	18g	Radix Scrophulariae

It was used tot treat 30 cases of stubborn urticaria with a total effectiveness rate of 100%. [17]

9) Wán Má Tāng (顽麻汤)

黄芪	huáng qí	20g	Radix Astragali
防风	fáng fēng	12g	Radix Saposhnikoviae
白鲜皮	bái xiān pí	12g	Cortex Dictamni
赤小豆	chì xiǎo dòu	15g	Semen Phaseoli
桂枝	guì zhī	15g	Ramulus Cinnamomi
当归	dāng guī	10g	Radix Angelicae Sinensis
白芍	bái sháo	10g	Radix Paeoniae Alba
川芎	chuān xiōng	10g	Rhizoma Chuanxiong
丹参	dān shēn	10g	Radix et Rhizoma Salviae Miltiorrhizae
红花	hóng huā	10g	Flos Carthami
僵蚕	jiāng cán	10g	Bombyx Batryticatus
苡仁	yǐ rén	10g	Semen Coicis
苍术	cāng zhú	10g	Rhizoma Atractylodis
乌梅	wū méi	10g	Fructus Mume
紫草	zǐ cǎo	10g	Radix Arnebiae
大青叶	dà qīng yè	10g	Folium Isatidis
五味子	wǔ wèi zǐ	10g	Fructus Schisandrae Chinensis
鸡血藤	jī xuè téng	10g	Caulis Spatholobi
生龙骨	shēng lóng gǔ	10g	Raw Os Draconis
酸枣仁	suān zǎo rén	10g	Semen Ziziphi Spinosae
生百部	shēng bǎi bù	10g	Raw Radix Stemonae
甘草	gān cǎo	10g	Radix et Rhizoma Glycyrrhizae
地肤子	dì fū zǐ	30g	Fructus Kochiae

It was used to treat 34 cases of chronic urticaria with 32 cases being cured and 2 cases receiving some effect.[18]

10) Yǎng Xuè Qū Fēng Tāng (养血祛风汤)

当归	dāng guī	15g	Radix Angelicae Sinensis
川芎	chuān xiōng	6g	Rhizoma Chuanxiong
赤芍	chì sháo	10g	Radix Paeoniae Rubra
荆芥	jīng jiè	10g	Herba Schizonepetae
防风	fáng fēng	10g	Radix Saposhnikoviae

生地	shēng dì	10g	Radix Rehmanniae Recens
玄参	xuán shēn	10g	Radix Scrophulariae
夜交藤	yè jiāo téng	10g	Caulis Polygoni Multiflori
麦冬	mài dōng	15g	Radix Ophiopogonis
白鲜皮	bái xiān pí	15g	Cortex Dictamni
土茯苓	tǔ fú líng	20g	Rhizoma Smilacis Glabrae

This formula was modified and used to treat 93 cases of urticaria with a total effectiveness rate of 92.7%. [19]

11) Xī Fēng Suān Méi Tāng (熄风酸梅汤)

荆芥	jīng jiè	12g	Herba Schizonepetae
丹参	dān shēn	12g	Radix et Rhizoma Salviae Miltiorrhizae
防风	fáng fēng	10g	Radix Saposhnikoviae
蝉衣	chán yī	10g	Periostracum Cicadae
乌梅	wū méi	10g	Fructus Mume
五味子	wǔ wèi zǐ	10g	Fructus Schisandrae Chinensis
甘草	gān cǎo	6g	Radix et Rhizoma Glycyrrhizae

It was used to treat 63 cases of chronic urticaria. The pattern that these cases belonged to was one of long-term Liver depression transforming into heat and damaging the yin. The total effectiveness rate was 92%. [20]

12) Yǐn Zhěn Tāng (瘾疹汤)

黄芪	huáng qí	20g	Radix Astragali
党参	dǎng shēn	20g	Radix Codonopsis
白鲜皮	bái xiān pí	15g	bái xiān pí
刺蒺藜	cì jí lí	15g	Fructus Tribuli
生地	shēng dì	15g	Radix Rehmanniae Recens
赤芍	chì sháo	12g	Radix Paeoniae Rubra
白芍	bái sháo	12g	Radix Paeoniae Alba
生首乌	shēng shǒu wū	10g	Raw Radix Polygoni Multiflori
当归	dāng guī	10g	Radix Angelicae Sinensis
川芎	chuān xiōng	10g	Rhizoma Chuanxiong

| 蝉蜕 | chán tuì | 10g | Periostracum Cicadae |
| 苦参 | kǔ shēn | 10g | Radix Sophorae Flavescentis |

It was used to treat 140 cases of chronic urticaria, with the formula modified according to the pattern. The curative rate was 50.71% and the total effectiveness rate was 83.57%. [21]

13) *Chái Cāng Jīng Chán Tāng* （柴苍荆蝉汤）

柴胡	chái hú	10g	Radix Bupleuri
苍术	cāng zhú	10g	Rhizoma Atractylodis
荆芥	jīng jiè	10g	Herba Schizonepetae
龙眼肉	lóng yǎn ròu	10g	Arillus Longan
蝉衣	chán yī	12	Periostracum Cicadae
威灵仙	wēi líng xiān	15g	Radix et Rhizoma Clematidis
红枣	hóng zǎo	4pieces	Fructus Jujubae
苏打粉	sū dǎ fěn	8g	soda powder

It was used to treat 200 cases of urticaria (with modifications to the formula), with a satisfying treatment effect. [22]

14) *Bái Shé Tāng* （白蛇汤）

白鲜皮	bái xiān pí	15g	Cortex Dictamni
蛇床子	shé chuáng zǐ	12g	Fructus Cnidii
百部	bǎi bù	12g	Radix Stemonae
荆芥	jīng jiè	10g	Herba Schizonepetae
防风	fáng fēng	10g	Radix Saposhnikoviae
薄荷	bò hé	10g	Herba Menthae
龙胆草	lóng dǎn cǎo	6g	Radix et Rhizoma Gentianae
蒲公英	pú gōng yīng	20g	Herba Taraxaci
苦参	kǔ shēn	15g	Radix Sophorae Flavescentis
黄柏	huáng bǎi	10g	Cortex Phellodendri Chinensis
全蝎	quán xiē	5g	Scorpio
蜈蚣	wú gōng	2pieces	Scolopendra
甘草	gān cǎo	5g	Radix et Rhizoma Glycyrrhizae

It was used to treat 46 cases of urticaria according to pattern differentiation. During the treatment, alcohol, spicy food, mutton, garlic and chives were prohibited. As a result, 40 cases were cured and 4 cases were alleviated. [23]

15) *Wŭ Zĭ Tāng* （五紫汤）

紫草	zĭ cǎo	30g	Radix Arnebiae
紫背浮萍	zĭ bèi fú píng	5g	Herba Spirodelae
紫花地丁	zĭ huā dì dīng	30g	Herba Violae
紫丹参	zĭ dān shēn	15g	Radix et Rhizoma Salviae Miltiorrhizae
紫贝齿	zĭ bèi chĭ	30g	Concha Cypraeae Violacae

The formula was particularly effective for stubborn urticatia. [24]

16) *Qí Píng Xiāo Yĭn Tāng* （芪萍消瘾汤）

生黄芪	shēng huáng qí		Raw Radix Astragali
党参	dǎng shēn		Radix Codonopsis
浮萍	fú píng		Herba Spirodelae
当归	dāng guī		Radix Angelicae Sinensis

It was used to treat 58 cases of chronic urticaria with a total effectiveness rate of 98.27%. [25]

17) Modified *Guì Zhī Er Má Huáng Yī Tāng* （桂枝二麻黄一汤） with *Táo Hóng Sì Wù Tāng* （桃红四物汤）

桂枝	guì zhī	12g	Ramulus Cinnamomi
当归	dāng guī	12g	Radix Angelicae Sinensis
麻黄	má huáng	6g	Herba Ephedrae
川芎	chuān xiōng	6g	Rhizoma Chuanxiong
红花	hóng huā	6g	Flos Carthami
炙甘草	zhì gān cǎo	6g	Radix et Rhizoma Glycyrrhizae Praeparata cum Melle
白芍	bái sháo	15g	Radix Paeoniae Alba
生地黄	shēng dì huáng	15g	Radix Rehmanniae Recens
威灵仙	wēi líng xiān	15g	Radix et Rhizoma Clematidis
生姜	shēng jiāng	9g	Rhizoma Zingiberis Recens

桃仁	táo rén	9g	Semen Persicae
防风	fáng fēng	9g	Radix Saposhnikoviae
蒺藜	jí lí	9g	Fructus Tribuli
乌梅	wū méi	9g	Fructus Mume
大枣	dà zǎo	7pieces	Fructus Jujubae

For bright red skin rashes with a burning sensation and severe pruritus, add *rěn dōng téng* (Caulis Lonicerae Japonicae) 30g and *mǔ dān pí* (Cortex Moutan) 12g.

For pale skin rashes aggravated by wind and cold, add *shēng huáng qí* (Raw Radix Astragali) 20g, and *bái zhú* (Rhizoma Atractylodis Macrocephalae) 12g.

For severe pruritus during the night, add *yè jiāo téng* (Caulis Polygoni Multiflori) 30g, and *chán tuì* (Periostracum Cicadae) 9g.

For skin rashes distributed mainly on the lower limbs, add *yì yǐ rén* (Semen Coicis) 30g, and *dì fū zǐ* (Fructus Kochiae) 15g.

For dry skin, add *hé shǒu wū* (Radix Polygoni Multiflori) 20g, and *gǒu qǐ zǐ* (Fructus Lycii) 15g. Decoct with water, take 1 dose every day, divided into two and consumed after meals. A course of treatment was one week. During the treatment other drugs and pungent and stimulating foods should be prohibited. As a result, 19 cases were cured, 10 cases were relieved and 3 cases show no effect. The clinical curing rate was 59.4% and the total effectiveness rate was 90.6%.[26]

18) *Kàng Mǐn Tāng* （抗敏汤）

何首乌	hé shǒu wū	15-25g	Radix Polygoni Multiflori
全当归	quán dāng guī	10-15g	Radix Angelicae Sinensis
白鲜皮	bái xiān pí	10-15g	Cortex Dictamni
丹皮	dān pí	10-15g	Cortex Moutan
乌蛇肉	wū shé ròu	10-15g	Zaocys
白僵蚕	bái jiāng cán	10-15g	Bombyx Batryticatus
蚕砂	cán shā	15-30g	Faeces Bombycis

Decoct with water and take 1 dose every day.

For exterior deficiency with wind, add *huáng qí* (Radix Astragali), and *fáng fēng* (Radix Saposhnikoviae).

For qi deficiency aggravated by fatigue, add *huáng qí* (Radix Astragali), and *dǎng shēn* (Radix Codonopsis).

For yang deficiency aggravated by cold, add *xiān líng pí* （Epimedium brevicornum Maxim), and *guì zhī* (Ramulus Cinnamomi).

For severe itching, add *quán xiē* (Scorpio), and *chán tuì* (Periostracum Cicadae).

It was used to treat 151 cases of chronic urticaria with a satisfying treatment effect. [27]

19) *Quán Chán Yǐn* （全蝉饮）

全蝎	quán xiē	3g	Scorpio
蝉蜕	chán tuì	10g	Periostracum Cicadae
僵蚕	jiāng cán	10g	Bombyx Batryticatus
防风	fáng fēng	10g	Radix Saposhnikoviae
秦艽	qín jiāo	10g	Radix Gentianae Macrophyllae
当归	dāng guī	10g	Radix Angelicae Sinensis
白芍	bái sháo	10g	Radix Paeoniae Alba

For a wind-heat pattern, add *jīn yín huā* (Flos Lonicerae Japonicae), *lián qiào* (Fructus Forsythiae), *mǔ dān pí* (Cortex Moutan), *chì sháo* (Radix Paeoniae Rubra), and *zǐ cǎo* (Radix Arnebiae).

For severe dampness add *xī xiān cǎo* (Herba Siegesbeckiae), *biǎn dòu* (Semen Lablab Album), and *fú líng* (Poria).

For insufficiency of both body fluids and blood, add *shēng dì* (Radix Rehmanniae Recens), *hé shǒu wū* (Radix Polygoni Multiflori), and *gǒu qǐ zǐ* (Fructus Lycii).

For qi deficiency, add *huáng qí* (Radix Astragali), and *bái zhú* （Rhizoma Atractylodis Macrocephalae).

For dry stool, add *huǒ má rén* (Fructus Cannabis) or *dà huáng* (Radix et Rhizoma Rhei).

It was used to treat 23 cases of urticaria. 12 cases were cured, 9 cases were relieved, and 2 cases showed no effect. The total effectiveness rate was 91.3% . [28]

3. ACUPUNCTURE AND MOXIBUSTION

(1) Body Acupuncture

Nie believes that the most common differentiation of chronic urticaria is cold and deficiency of the Spleen and Stomach, so mild moxibustion should be used. He chose CV 8 (*shéng quē*), and ST 36 (*zú sān lǐ*) to do moxibustion for ten minutes daily. Ten times is a therapeutic course. 18 cases received this treatment and all of them were cured[29].

Yang Xin-jing applied an herbal paste on acupuncture points to treat chronic urticaria. The herbs used were:

党参	dǎng shēn	20g	Radix Codnopsis
黄芪	huáng qí	20g	Radix Astragali
紫草	zǐ cǎo	20g	Radix Arnebiae
知母	zhī mǔ	20g	Rhizoma Anemarrhenae
大黄	dà huáng	20g	Radix et Rhizoma Rhei
郁金	yù jīn	15g	Radix Curcumae
赤芍	chì sháo	15g	Radix Paeoniae Rubra
白术	bái zhú	15g	Rhizoma Atractylodis Macrocephalae
石膏	shí gāo	15g	Gypsum Fibrosum
甘草	gān cǎo	10g	Radix et Rhizoma Glycyrrhizae

He ground these into powder and mixed the powder with ginger juice. Then he cut a slice of mixed herbs about 0.5 cm thick, and fixed it on the acupuncture points with a piece of adhesive plaster.

The main points used were:

LI 4	hé gǔ	合谷
LI 11	qū chí	曲池
SP 10	xuè hǎi	血海
DU 14	dà zhuī	大椎

From which 2 to 3 points were selected per treatment. The course of treatment was 7 days, one treatment per day. He treated 287 cases with a total effectiveness rate of 95.8% [30].

Wang Yuan believes that urticaria should be treated by coursing wind, clearing heat, and harmonizing *ying*. Pricking cupping can be used to drain accumulations of damp heat toxic evils in the channel sinews and skin.

Main points:

DU 14	dà zhuī	大椎
LI 11	qū chí	曲池
LI 4	hé gǔ	合谷
SP 10	xuè hǎi	血海
GB 20	fēng chí	风池

Adjunctive points:

HT 7	shén mén	神门
SP 9	yīn líng quán	阴陵泉

DU 14 (*dà zhuī*)) located on the Governing Vessel (which controls the *yang qi* of the entire body), was the main point for reducing heat. Pricking cupping on DU 14 (*dà zhuī*)) can discharge blood so as to clear heat. GB 20 (*fēng chí*) was used to course wind and clear heat; LI 11 (*qū chí*) and LI 4 (*hé gǔ*) were used to clear heat in the *Yangming* channel and harmonize ying and wei. SP 10 (*xuè hǎi*) was used to regulate qi and blood, clear heat, and remove dampness. This combination of four points can course wind and clear heat, invigorate the blood and harmonize the *ying*. These are the major points to treat urticaria caused by wind-heat. HT 7 (*shén mén*) calms the mind and stops itching, while SP 9 (*yīn líng quán*) drains dampness and clears heat. The combination of all of the above points can course wind, clear heat, invigorate blood, and stop itching. After sterilization, apply pricking cupping on DU 14 (*dà zhuī*)), discharging 5-10 milliliters of blood. Then needle perpendicularly, 0.5 to 1 cun deep and manipulate to drain by lifting and thrusting the needle on LI 4 (*hé gǔ*), and SP 10 (*xuè hǎi*). This technique is carried out for one minute. Then drain GB 20 (*fēng chí*) by twirling and rotating the needle after inserting it perpendicularly 0.5 cun. This is also done for one minute. The needle retention was twenty minutes. HT 7 (*shén mén*) and SP 9 (*yīn líng quán*) were needled perpendicularly using a draining twirling and rotating manipulation. At the same time, the following were prohibited – a stimulating diet, fish, and exposure to wind when sweating or after bathing.

Song Yu-hua treated 38 cases of chronic stubborn urticaria with acupuncture. According to pattern differentiation, the disease was divided into the following categories: wind-evil invading the exterior, Stomach and Intestine damp heat, and blood dryness engendering wind.

There were four groups of points combination.

Group 1:

BL 40	wěi zhōng	委中
LU 5	chǐ zé	尺泽

The points were pricked with a three-edged needle to discharge blood in order to clear heat in the blood level. 5-6 drops of blood were let each time.

Group 2:

LI 11	qū chí	曲池
SP 10	xuè hǎi	血海
GB 31	fēng shì	风市
SJ 5	wài guān	外关

BL 17	gé shū	膈俞
BL 12	fēng mén	风门
BL 13	fèi shū	肺俞

The points were needled with a rotating draining technique so as to course wind and harmonize *ying*. For each treatment 3-4 points were chosen, alternating the points each time. The needles were retained for 20 minutes each treatment.

Group 3:

RN 12	zhōng wǎn	中脘
ST 25	tiān shū	天枢
SP 6	sān yīn jiāo	三阴交
ST 36	zú sān lǐ	足三里
SP 4	gōng sūn	公孙

The points were needled with an even supplementation and drainage method for twenty minutes so as to regulate the Middle Jiao and invigorate the Spleen and Stomach.

Group 4:

KI 16	zhào hǎi	照海
BL 23	shèn shū	肾俞
BL 18	gān shū	肝俞
BL 20	pí shū	脾俞

The points were needled with a supplementing rotating technique so as to tonify the Kidneys, boost qi, soften the Liver, fortify the Spleen, nourish blood, harmonize blood, moisten dryness, and stop itching. The above four sets of points have different functions and indications. The first three groups were used daily to treat acute attacks of chronic urticaria caused by wind-evil invading the exterior or damp-heat in the Stomach and the Intestines. The latter three groups were used for the chronic urticaria caused by damp-heat in the Stomach and the Intestines or blood dryness engendering wind. Ten treatments was a therapeutic course. A three-to- five day break was suggested during two therapeutic courses. The total effectiveness rate was 97.4%.

Chen Zhi-xing treated urticaria with acupuncture. 153 cases were divided randomly into 108 cases in the acupuncture treatment group and 45 cases in the control group.

For the control group, the points combination were:

LI 11	qū chí	曲池
LI 4	hé gǔ	合谷
ST 36	zú sān lǐ	足三里
SP 10	xuè hǎi	血海
SP 6	sān yīn jiāo	三阴交
LE 3	bǎi chóng wō	百虫窝
GB 34	yáng líng quán	阳陵泉
GB 20	fēng chí	风池
DU 14	dà zhuī	大椎

Two to three points were punctured daily, and this constituted one treatment. Ten treatments were a theraputic course. Teldane (60 mg) and Vitamin C (200 mg or a half dose for children) were taken orally by patients in the control group. Other anti-allergy and anti-itching medications were forbidden during the two-week study. The final total effectiveness rate was 65.7% for the acupuncture treatment group, and 46.7% for the control group.

Liu Guo-xiang treated 45 cases of urticaria.

1) Points on the hand *Yangming* and foot *Taiyin* channels were chosen.

A drainage technique with filiform needles was used.

LI 11 (*qū chí*), SP 10 (*xuè hǎi*), and LI 4 (*hé gǔ*), were selected as the chief points,

Main points:

LI 11	qū chí	曲池
SP 10	xuè hǎi	血海
LI 4	hé gǔ	合谷

Adjunctive points:

ST 36	zú sān lǐ	足三里
LV 3	tài chōng	太冲
GB 20	fēng chí	风池

DU 14 (*dà zhuī*) was pricked with a three-edged needle and then cupped for ten minutes so as to expel wind-evil and clear heat in blood.

2) Points on Bladder channel of the foot *Taiyang* were chosen as the chief points.

Such as BL 17 (*gé shū*), BL 20 (*pí shū*) and BL 21 (*wèi shū*).

Main points:

BL 17	gé shū	膈俞
BL 20	pí shū	脾俞
BL 21	wèi shū	胃俞

Adjunctive points:

| BL 40 | wěi zhōng | 委中 |
| SJ 10 | tiān jǐng | 天井 |

They were needled with an even supplementation and drainage technique so as to clear toxins and heat in the blood. The total effectiveness rate was 80% [34].

Shi Li-yan treated 45 cases of urticaria by bleeding cupping.

Points combination:

DU 14	dà zhuī	大椎
BL 13	fèi shū	肺俞
BL 25	dà cháng shū	大肠俞

The method was as followed: lying in a prone posture, after routine sterilization, the patients were swiftly pricked by a two-edged needle followed by 5 minutes of cupping until the point bled. This was done one time a day. 3 times was a therapeutic course. The total effectiveness rate was 100% [35].

Zhang Chun-jing used bleeding cupping to treat urticaria. The Governing vessel, *Jiá Jí* points, and *Taiyang* channel were tapped from upper part to lower part using a seven-star needle. There was an emphasis on the neck, the *positive* areas, GB 20 (*fēng chí*), DU 14 (*dà zhuī*) and LI 11 (*qū chí*). These were tapped heavily until there was slight bleeding, then cups were applied on the areas. BL 18 (*gān shū*), and BL 17 (*gé shū*) were recommended to be heavily pricked for cases of chronic urticaria. Liu Ying also reported treating 103 cases of measles by cupping on RN 8 (*shén quē*). The total effectiveness rate was 97.1%.

(2) Scalp Acupuncture

Mo Xiao-feng treated 40 cases of chronic urticaria with scalp acupuncture. He selected the first line of the forehead (bilaterally), the lateral line of the vertex-temporal line (bilaterally), and the middle line of the forehead. He used 1.5 cun long #32 needles to needle the scalp at an angle of 30 degrees between the needle and the scalp. The needles were swiftly inserted into the lower level of the epicranial aponeurosis, then turned horizontally for complete needling. The depth of insertion was 1-1.2 cun. Needles were rotated 200 times a minute for 1-2 minutes. After the qi arrived, the patients were told to relax with their eyes closed, imagining the qi reaching the skin. The doctor concentrated on the tips of the needles. For the first and middle lines of the forehead, the needle was inserted from the upper part to the lower part. For lateral line of the vertex-temporal line, 3-4 needles were used in a line. The retention time was 1 hour. One treatment was done every two days and 10 treatments were a therapeutic course. Between the two therapeutic courses, a three day break was taken. The treatment effect was observed after two therapeutic courses. The total effectiveness rate was 100 %[38].

(3) Auricular Acupuncture

Wang An selected following auricular points:

ear apex	EX-HN6	ěr jiān	耳尖
ear center	HX1	ěr zhōng	耳中
wind stream	SF1	fēng xī	风溪
endocrine	CO18	nèi fēn mì	内分泌
lung of posterior surface	P2	ěr bèi fèi	耳背肺
spleen of posterior surface	P3	ěr bèi pǐ	耳背脾
large intestine	CO6	dà cháng	大肠
occiput	AT3	zhěn	枕
adrenal gland	TG2p	shèn shàng xiàn	肾上腺

Each point was covered with a piece of adhesive with a *wang bu liu xing* (Semen Vaccariae) seed on it. The patients were asked to press the seeds fifteen times with their thumb and index finger, three times a day. Each side was used alternately every other day. Ten times was a therapeutic course. It got an outstanding treatment effect [39].

Zhao Yong-zhou selected following auricular points:

shen men	TF4	shén mén	神门
heart	CO15	xīn	心
lung of posterior surface	P2	ěr bèi fèi	耳背肺
anti-allergic region		kàng guò mǐn qū	抗过敏区
sebaceous gland		pí zhǐ xiàn	皮脂腺
spleen of posterior surface	P3	ěr bèi pǐ	耳背脾
stomach	CO4	wèi	胃
ear apex	EX-HN6	ěr jiān	耳尖

Points were modified in accordance with symptoms to treat urticaria. The points were covered with an adhesive with *Wang bu liu xing* (Semen

Vaccariae) seads, and pressed twice a day. Five to ten treatments was a therapeutic course. The opposite side was used fifteen days after a course of treatment. Seven courses of treatment were given, on average, to 121 patients. Among them 35 were cured, 41 showed obvious treatment effect, 34 had some treatment effect and 11 had no treatment effect [40].

Shi Cheng-ming treated 86 cases of chronic urticaria with bleeding pricking on auricular points. He chose the urticaria region on one side of the ear (the space between fingers and wrist on the Scaphoid fossa) and made a moderately deep cut about 2 cm long (the auricular cartilage was not damaged) by using a sterilized operating knife blade. Three to four drops of blood were squeezed out before the cut was covered by a piece of sterilized gauze and adhesive tape. The other ear was used one week later. Seven treatments was a therapeutic course, with the opposite ear used every other time. 52 cases were cured[41].

Yang Xi-sen treated 50 cases of chronic urticaria with auricular pressure methods. He chose the urticaria region as the chief point, and the endocrine region as the secondary point. Both sides were sterilized and then covered by a 0.6 mm X 0.6 mm plaster with *Wang bu liu xing* (Semen Vaccariae) seeds. The points were pressed (with the fingers) three to four times a day. The plasters were changed every three to five days. Seven treatments were a therapeutic course. 48 cases were cured, and 2 cases stopped treatment early due to other diseases [42].

Experimental Studies

1. RESEARCH ON THE EFFICACY OF SINGLE CHINESE MEDICINALS

(1) Experimental studies of *Léi Gōng Téng* （雷公藤）tablets to treat chronic urticaria

Li Xing-wen divided 64 cases of chronic urticaria into two groups. For the treatment group, *Lei Gong Teng* tablets were given orally, one tablet a time, three times a day. For the control group Cyproheptadine was given orally, 2 mg each time, 3 times a day. One month was a course of treatment. The result showed that the total effectiveness rate for *Lei Gong Teng* tablet was 97% - obviously higher than the 83.3% for the control group. Pharmacological experiments revealed that the main component of *Lei Gong Teng* tablets was *Lei Gong Teng* polyglycoside which has strong anti-inflammatory and immunosuppressive functions. It can have hormone-like actions, but without the side effects of hormones. It competes with the histamine receptor on mast cells so as to prevent the release of histamine for a longer time, and reduce capillary permeability. These functions help to treat urticaria[43].

(2) *Yún Nán Bái Yào*（云南白药）

Yún Nán Bái Yào is a commonly used coagulant. It contains saponins which have significant anti-inflammatory effects. It can promote the secretion of corticosteroids, restrain the media release of the inflammatory process, and increase capillary permeability, thereby treating urticaria. Huang Zhi-jian treated 29 cases of chronic urticaria by orally administering *Yún Nán Bái Yào*. The total effectiveness rate was 90.62%[44].

(3) *Yì mǔ cǎo* (Herba Leonuri)

Yì mǔ cǎo is pungent and sweet in flavor, slightly cold in property, and has the functions of moving blood and removing blood stasis, reducing edema, promoting urination, clearing heat and resolving toxin. Used orally or as a wash, it can remove allergens, act as an antihistamine, and improve blood flow of the skin. It was recorded in the *Divine Husbandman's Classic of Meteria Medica* (神农本草经 , *Shén Nóng Běn Cǎo Jīng*) that *yì mǔ cǎo* (Herba Leonuri) can be used to treat insidious rashes. Cai Wen-ke used it both orally and externally to treat 30 cases of urticaria. All of them received effect[45].

(4) *Fáng fēng* (Radix Saposhnikoviae) and *cì jí lí* (Fructus Tribuli)

Fáng fēng (Radix Saposhnikoviae) and *cì jí lí* (Fructus Tribuli) combined and fried together can stop itching in animal model experiments. In these animal models, pruritus was caused by exogenous histamines and endogenous histamines induced by dextran. This combination also can restrain the increased capillary permeability caused by histamine. It can also, to some degree, restrain the swelling of guinea pig ears as induced by dimethyl sulphoxide. This reveals that the combination of *fáng fēng* (Radix Saposhnikoviae) and *cì jí lí* (Fructus Tribuli) has an anti-allergic effect. The combination of *fáng fēng* (Radix Saposhnikoviae) with *cì jí lí* (Fructus Tribuli) is more effective than either herb used alone[46].

2. RESEARCH ON THE EFFICACY OF HERBAL PRESCRIPTIONS

1) *Guī Pí Wán* （归脾丸） treats chronic urticaria :

Han Zi-ying used *Guī Pí Wán* orally to treat 42 cases of chronic urticaria. The treatment was 1 tablet per dose, twice a day. Ten days was a course of treatment, with a total of 5-6 courses. The curative rate was 71.4% and the total effectiveness rate was 83.3%. Research revealed that *Guī Pí Wán* tonifies qi, nourishes blood, strengthens the Spleen, and nourishes the Heart. It can restrain the production of IgE antibodies, enhance cellular immune function, adjust the ratio of intestinal flora, and promote SIGA secretion, thereby creating mucous membrane barriers to prevent allergen factors from entering into the blood. It had a satisfying effect to treat chronic urticaria[47].

2) *Qīng Rè Qū Fēng Chōng Jì* （清热祛风冲剂） treats wind heat urticaria:

Ding Su-fu used *Qīng Rè Qū Fēng Chōng Jì* (*jīng jiè* [Herba Schizonepetae], *fáng fēng* [Radix Saposhnikoviae], *huáng qín* [Radix

Scutellariae], *lián qiào* [Fructus Forsythiae], *huáng bǎi* [Cortex Phellodendri Chinensis], *kǔ shēn* [Radix Sophorae Flavescentis], *bái xiān pí* [Cortex Dictamni], *shēng dì* [Radix Rehmanniae Recens], and *gān cǎo* [Radix et Rhizoma Glycyrrhizae]) to treat acute and chronic urticaria. The effectiveness rate for 167 cases of acute urticaria was 88.8% and for chronic cases it was 50%. Clinical pharmacological tests showed that it can control inflammation, effusion and allergic reactions. Individual herbs in the prescription have anti-allergic, antipyretic and anti-inflammatory effects. Thereby this formula can treat type I allergic skin disease well [48].

3) *Yù Píng Fēng Sǎn* treats chronic urticaria:

Chen Hong used *Yù Píng Fēng Sǎn* to treat chronic urticaria. The curative rate was 27.3%, the total effectiveness rate was 77.3% and the reoccurrence rate after stopping the treatment was 28.8%. In addition, the patients' IgE blood serum level had significantly decreased. These effectiveness rates are significantly different than the control group, which was treated with biomedicine[49].

4) *Dāng Guī Yǐn Zi* treats chronic urticaria:

Xiao Hong-li used *Dāng Guī Yǐn Zī* to treat chronic urticaria. The reoccurrence rate and time between reoccurrences in the treatment group were superior to those in the control group (which was treated with Loratadine). After the treatment, the patients who originally had increased IgE rates had lower rates. *Dāng Guī Yǐn Zī* can also increase T lymphocyte transformation[50].

3. RESEARCH ON ACUPUNCTURE MECHANISM

Che Jian-li discussed the influence of acupuncture on IgE blood serum levels in patients with chronic urticaria. Immune parameters were observed to be dynamic in many stages of the disease, both before and after acupuncture treatment. The results showed that patients with chronic urticaria had higher IgE levels than healthy people, and acupuncture for chronic urticaria patients had positive IgE regulation. Thereby it confirmed that acupuncture had positive regulating functions for these kinds of patients [51].

Song Chun-hua and others observed the treatment effect of acupuncture on chronic urticaria patients. LI 11 (*qū chí*) was needled bilaterally in the treatment group and Cetirizine was given orally in the control group. Comparison of the treatment effects in the two groups looked at the quantity and size of the skin rashes, the degree of pruritus, and the number of flare-ups. The results showed that after treatments the two groups had significant differences in rash quality and size, degree of pruritus, and the number of flare ups within one week (P<0.01). The acupuncture group was superior to the biomedicine group in improvements of the above parameters (P<0.01). The two groups had significant differences in the curative effect (P<0.01) [52].

REFERENCES

[1] Xuan Guo-wei. Treatment According to Traditional Chinese Medicine Syndrome Differentiation of Chronic Urticaria (慢性荨麻疹的中医辨证治疗). *The Journal of Practical Medicine* (实用医学杂志),1991, 7(5)：260

[2] Fan Rui-qiang, Xie Chang-cai. The Experience of Treating Chronic Urticaria by Professor. Xuan Guo-wei (禤国维教授治疗慢性荨麻疹的经验). *Traditional Chinese Medicine Study* (中医药研究), 1999,(5)：15

[3] Chen Da-can, Liu Ai-min. Samples of Professor. Xuan Guo-wei's Experience of Treating Difficult Skin Diseases by Tonifying the Kidney (禤国维教授运用补肾法治疗疑难皮肤病经验举隅). *Shanghai Journal of Traditional Chinese Medicine* (上海中医药杂志), 2004 38(2)：39

[4] Zheng Wei-qin. The Summary of Old TCM Doctor Zhou Bai-chuan's Experience

of Treating Urticaria (老中医周百川治疗荨麻疹经验总结). *Yunnan Journal of Traditional Chinese Medicine* (云南中医药杂志), 1997, 18(2)：32

[5] E Yong-an. Samples of Zhu Liang-chun's Experience In Treating Skin Diseases (朱良春论治皮肤病经验举要). *Sichuan Journal of Traditional Chinese Medicine* (四川中医) ,2003, 21(10)：3

[6] Xu Wen-jun. Zhang Zuo-zhou's Experience In Treating Refractory Urticaria (张作舟治疗顽固性荨麻疹经验). *China's Naturopathy* (中国民间疗法), 1998,(3)：32

[7] Zhao Pei-ling, Gong Guo-mu-liang. Treating 26 Cases of Urticaria According to Syndrome Differentiation (辨证治疗荨麻疹26例). *Beijing Journal of Traditional Chinese Medicine* (北京中医药), 1996,(4)：6

[8] Liu Gui-jun, Wang Yu-xi. Prof. Wang Yu-xi's Experience In Treating Urticaria

[9] Shi Xin. Shi Guan-qing's Experience In Treating Chronic Urticaria According to Syndrome Differentiation (石冠卿辨证治疗慢性荨麻疹经验). *Shandong Journal of Traditional Chinese Medicine* (山东中医杂志), 2005, 24(3)：176

[10] Li Zhi-xia. Treating Urticaria with *Wu she Chan Tui* Decoction (乌蛇蝉蜕汤治疗荨麻疹). *Shandong Journal of Traditional Chinese Medicine* (山东中医杂志), 2003, 22 (8)：461

[11] Wang Yu-zhen, Liu Jian-ping, et al. Treating 60 Cases of Wind-Heat Acute Urticaria by *Qu Qian* Decoction (祛荨汤治疗风热型急性荨麻疹60例). *Hebei Journal of Traditional Chinese Medicine* (河北中医),1995,17(3)：40

[12] Li Zhi-zhen, Sun Wei. Treating Refractory Urticaria From Weakened Defensive *Wei* Syndrome by *Gubiao Qufeng* Decoction (固表祛风汤治疗卫表不固型顽固性荨麻疹). *Jiangxi Journal of Traditional Chinese Medicine* (江西中医药), 2001, 32(6)：37

[13] Li Rui-kun, Zheng Feng-lan, etc. Observations of Treating 72 Cases of Urticaria with Chinese Herbs (中药治疗荨麻疹72例观察). *Hebei Journal of Traditional Chinese Medicine* (河北中医), 1996, 18(3)：10

[14] He Ying-kun. Summary of Treating 178 Cases of Urticaria with *Jinfang Siwu* Decoction (荆防四物汤治疗荨麻疹178例总结). *Hunan Guiding Journal of Traditional Chinese Medicine and Pharmacology* (湖南中医药导报), 2001, 7(8)：410

[15] Zhang Yun-ping. Observation of 66 Cases of Chronic Urticaria Treated with *Huoxue Qufeng* Decoction (活血祛风汤治疗慢性荨麻疹66例疗效观察). *The Chinese Journal of Dermatovenereology* (中国皮肤性病学杂志), 2005, 19(4):243

[16] Zhang Shen-shu, Zhu Xiao-jun. Treating 46 Cases of Refractory Urticaria with *Jia Wei Tuo Min* Decoction (脱敏汤加味治疗顽固性荨麻疹46例). *Journal of Practical Traditional Chinese Medicine* (实用中医药杂志), 1997,(6)：12

[17] Jin Zhi-dao. Treating Refractory Urticaria with *Xiao Zhen* Decoction (消疹饮治疗顽固性荨麻疹). *Hubei Journal of Traditional Chinese Medicine* (湖北中医杂志), 1996, 18(60)：26

[18] Li Cai-xia. Treating 34 Cases of Chronic Urticaria with *Wan Ma* Decoction (顽麻汤治疗慢性荨麻疹34例). *Shaanxi Journal of Traditional Chinese Medicine* (陕西中医), 1997, 18(10)：464

[19] Wei Wu-jie. Treating 93 Cases of Chronic Urticaria with *Yangxue Qufeng* Decoction (养血祛风汤治疗慢性荨麻疹93例). *Hebei Journal of Traditional Chinese Medicine* (河北中医),2002,24(5)：339

[20] Zhang Xi-xiang. Treating 63 Cases of Chronic Urticaria with *Xifeng Suanmei* Decoction (熄风酸梅汤治疗慢性荨麻疹63例). *Shaanxi Journal of Traditional Chinese Medicine* (*Shan Xi Zhong Yi*) 陕西中医, 1997,(10)：465

[21] Guo Yu-qin. Observation of Treating 140 Cases of Chronic Urticaria with *Yin Zhen* Decoction (瘾疹汤治疗慢性荨麻疹140例观察). *Beijing Journal of Traditional Chinese Medicine* (北京中医), 2001, 4：16

[22] Huang Jia-chi, Li Guo-fu. Treating 200 Cases of Urticaria with *Chai Cang Jin Chan* Decoction (柴苍荆蝉汤治疗荨麻疹200例). *Journal of Practical Traditional Chinese Medicine* (实用中医药杂志), 2003, 19(10)：518

[23] He Jing-lin, Chen Shi-xiu,. Treating Refractory Urticaria with *Baishe* Decoction (白蛇汤治疗顽固性荨麻疹). *Journal of Chinese Physician* (中国临床医生), 2003,31(2)：27

[24] Guo Ling. Practice of Treating Refractory Urticaria with *Wu Zi* Decoction (五紫汤治疗顽固性荨麻疹实践). *Laser Journal* (激光杂志), 2003, 24(4)：35

[25] Du Zhi-qin ,Xu Ming-shou, Yang Chuan-wen. Treating 58 Cases of Chronic Urticaria with *Qi Ping Xiao Yin* Decoction (芪萍消瘾汤治疗慢性荨麻疹58例). *Shaanxi Journal of Traditional Chinese Medicine* (陕西中医), 2003, 24(9)：792

[26] Zhou Hai-hong. Observation of Treating 32 Cases of Chronic Urticaria with *Guizhi Er Mahuang Yi* Decoction Together with *Tao Hong Si Wu* Decoction (桂枝二麻黄一汤合桃红四物汤治疗慢性荨麻疹32例疗效观察). *New Journal of Traditional Chinese Medicine* (新中医), 2004, 36(5)：47

[27] Li Gui-qiang, Li Yun-zhu. Treating 42 Cases of Refractory Urticaria with *Kang Min* Decoction (抗敏汤治疗顽固性荨麻疹42例). *Shaanxi Journal of Traditional Chinese Medicine* (陕西中医), 2004, 25(3)：253

[28] Guo Lin-sheng. Treating 23 Cases of Urticaria with *Quan Chan* Decoction (全蝉饮治疗荨麻疹23例). *Jilin Journal of Traditional Chinese Medicine* (吉林中医药), 2005, 25(2)：24

[29] Nie Xi-jun. Treating 18 Cases of Chronic Urticaria by Moxibustion (艾灸治疗慢性荨麻疹18例). *Journal of Practical Traditional Chinese Medicine* (实用中医药杂志), 1992, (1)：40

[30] Yang Xin-jing. Treating 287 Cases of Chronic Urticaria by Adhering Herbs onto Acupuncture Points (中药贴穴治疗慢性荨麻疹287例). *Chinese Journal of Dermatology* (中华皮肤科杂志), 1991,(3)173

[31] Wang Yuan. Treating 32 Cases of Chronic Urticaria with Acupuncture (针刺治疗慢性荨麻疹32例). *Shanghai Journal of Acupuncture and Moxibustion* (上海针灸杂志), 2005, 24(5)：18

[32] Song Yu-hua, Wang Meng, Chen Quan. Treating Chronic and Refractory Urticaria with Acupuncture (针刺治疗慢性顽固性荨麻疹). *Chinese Acupuncture and Moxibustion* (中国针灸) , 2000 , 20 (12)：759

[33] Chen Zhi-xing, Zhao Xiao-wei, Sun Ying. Treating Urticaria with Acupuncture (针刺疗法治疗荨麻疹) *China's Naturopathy* 中国民间疗法, 2002, 10(5)：15 – 16

[34] Liu Guo-xiang, Jia Gui-zhi. Treating Urticaria with Acupuncture and Moxibustion (针灸治疗荨麻疹). *Heilongjiang Medicine and Pharmacy* (黑龙江医药科学),

2001，24 (3)：115

[35] Shi Li-yan. Treating Urticaria with Bleeding Cupping (刺血拔罐法治疗荨麻疹). *Chinese Acuponcture and Moxibustion* (中国针灸), 2000, 20(12)：760

[36] Zhang Chun-jing. Clinical Application of Blood-letting Therapy with Plum Needle (絮刺火罐疗法的临床运用) *Journal of Clinical Acupuncture and Moxibustion* (针灸临床杂志), 2002, 18 (1)：37 – 38

[37] Liu Ying, Wu Lan, Cui Jing. Treating 103 Cases of Acute Urticaria by Cupping *Shenque* (神阙穴拔火罐治疗急性荨麻疹103例). *Neimenggu Journal of Traditional Chinese Medicine* (内蒙古中医药), 2001 ,20(3)：28

[38] Mo Xiao-feng. Treating 40 Cases of Chronic Urticaria with Scalp Acupuncture (头皮针治疗慢性荨麻疹40例). *Zhejiang Journal of Traditional Chinese Medicine* (浙江中医杂志), 2002 ,37 (8)：360

[39] Wang An-jun. Treating 86 Cases of Urticaria with Auricular Herbal Seed Therapy (耳穴贴压法治疗荨麻疹86例). *Heilongjiang Journal of Traditional Chinese Medicine* (黑龙江中医药) ,2003,(1)：46

[40] Zhao Yong-zhou. Treating 121 Cases of Urticaria with Auricular Herbal Seed Therapy (耳穴贴压治疗荨麻疹121例). *Chinese Acuponcture and Moxibustion* (中国针灸), 1993,(1)：27

[41] Shi Cheng-min, Gao Li etc. Treating 86 Cases of Chronic Urticaria by Auricular Cutting Therapy (耳穴割治治疗慢性荨麻疹86例). *Li Shizhen Medicine and Medica Research* (时珍国医国药) ,2000,(9)：32

[42] Yang Xi-sen, Wang Cheng-guo. Treating 50 Cases of Chronic Urticaria by Auricular Herbal Seed Therapy (耳穴贴压治疗慢性荨麻疹 50 例) *Chinese Acupuncture and Moxibustion* (中国针灸) ,2002 ,22(2) :131

[43] Li Xing-wen. Treating 34 Cases of Chronic Urticaria with *Leigongteng* Pills (雷公藤片治疗慢性荨麻疹34例). *Journal of Clinical Dermatology* (临床皮肤科杂志), 1994, 23 (1)： 54

[44] Cai Wen-ke, Shi Zhang-ying. Treating Urticaria with *Leonurus Heterophyllus* (益母草治疗荨麻疹). *Zhejiang Journal of Traditional Chinese Medicine* (浙江中医杂志), 2001, 1(2)：159

[45] Huang Zhi-jian. Treating 32 Cases of Urticaria with *Yunnan Bai Yao* Powder (云南白药治疗荨麻疹32例). *Guangxi Journal of Traditional Chinese Medicine* (广西中医药), 1989, 12(3)：20

[46] Chen Zi-jun, Li Qing-sheng, Li Yun-sen, et al. Pharmacodynamics Study on Radix saposhnikoviae (RL) and Feutus tribuli (FI) (防风与刺蒺藜的药理实验研究). *Chinese Traditional Patent Medicine* (中成药), 2003, 25(9)：737

[47] Han Zi-ying, Wang Yu-zhen, et al. Treating 42 Cases of Chronic Urticaria with *Gui Pi Pill* (归脾丸治疗慢性荨麻疹42例). *The Chinese Journal of Dermatovenereology* (中国皮肤性病学杂志)，1997, 11(5)：294

[48] Ding Su-xian, Kuang Pu, et al. Clinical Observation and Pharmacodynamics Study of Treating Urticaria and Eczema with *Qingre Qufeng* Medicinal Instant Granules (清热祛风冲剂治疗荨麻疹、湿疹临床观察与药理实验). *The Chinese Journal of Dermatovenereology* (中国皮肤性病学杂志)，1994, 8(4)：247

[49] Chen Hong, Guo Yu-nan. Clinical Observation of Treating Chronic Urticaria with *Yu Ping Feng* Powder and Its Effect on Blood Serum IgE Levels (玉屏风散治疗慢性荨麻疹的临床观察及其对血清IgE水平的影响). *Journal of Chinese Medicinal Materials* (中药材), 2003,(2)：151

[50] Xiao Hong-li, Chen Han-zhang. Clinical Observation of Treating Chronic Urticaria with *Danggui Yinzi* (当归饮子治疗慢性荨麻疹的临床观察). *Sichuan Journal of Traditional Chinese Medicine* (四川中医), 2002, 20 (1)：62

[51] Che Jian-li. Clinical Study of the Effect of Acupuncture on the Blood Serum IgE Levels of Chronic Urticaria Patients (针刺对慢性荨麻疹患者血清IgE水平影响的临床研究). *Shandong Journal of Traditional Chinese Medicine* (山东中医杂志), 2005, 24(3)：158

[52] Song Chun-hua, Dong Gui-rong, Yang Su-qing, et al. Clinical Observation of Treating Chronic Urticaria by Puncturing *Quchi* (曲池穴针刺治疗慢性荨麻疹的临床观察) *Acupuncture and Moxibustion* (上海针灸杂志), 2005, 24(8)：17

Index by Disease Names and Symptoms

Index by Chinese Medicinals and Formulas

General Index

图书在版编目（CIP）数据

中医临床实用系列：荨麻疹（英文）/ 卢传坚等主编.
—北京：人民卫生出版社，2007.3
ISBN 978-7-117-08533-5

Ⅰ. 中⋯　Ⅱ. 卢⋯　Ⅲ. 荨麻诊 — 中医治疗法 — 英文
Ⅳ. R275.982.4

中国版本图书馆 CIP 数据核字（2007）第 024376 号

中医临床实用系列：荨麻疹（英文）

主　　编：卢传坚　陈达灿
出版发行：人民卫生出版社（中继线 +8610-6761-6688）
地　　址：中国北京丰台区方庄芳群园三区 3 号楼
邮　　编：100078
网　　址：http://www.pmph.com
E - mail：pmph @ pmph.com
发　　行：zzg@pmph.com.cn
购书热线：+8610-6769-1034（电话及传真）
开　　本：787×1092　1/16
版　　次：2007 年 3 月第 1 版　2007 年 3 月第 1 版第 1 次印刷
标准书号：ISBN 978-7-117-08533-5/R·8534